Essential Oil
RECIPES

FOR HOME AND BODY CARE

ISBN 978-1-4971-0333-7

Library of Congress Control Number: 2023935680

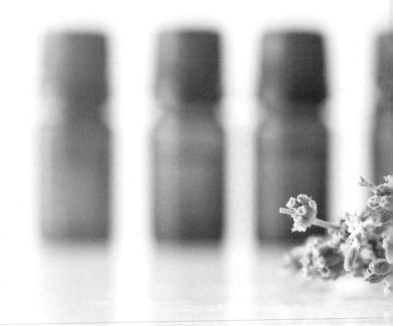

To learn more about the other great books from Fox Chapel Publishing, or to find a retailer near you, call toll-free 800-457-9112 or visit us at *www.FoxChapelPublishing.com*.

We are always looking for talented authors. To submit an idea, please send a brief inquiry to acquisitions@foxchapelpublishing.com.

Printed in China
First printing

Essential Oil RECIPES

100+

ORGANIC PRODUCTS
TO HELP YOU FEEL BETTER

Stephanie Ariel

TABLE OF
Contents

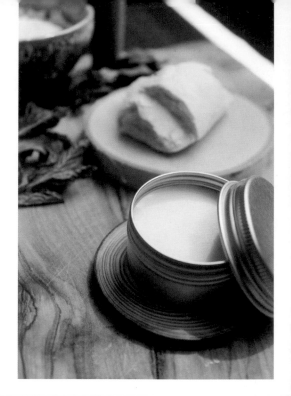

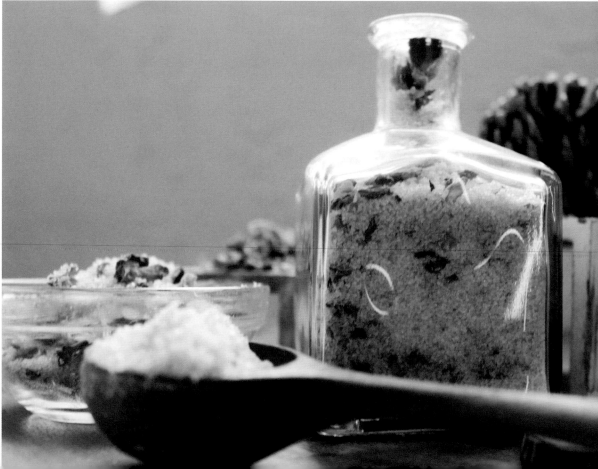

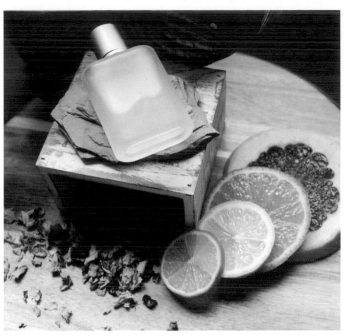

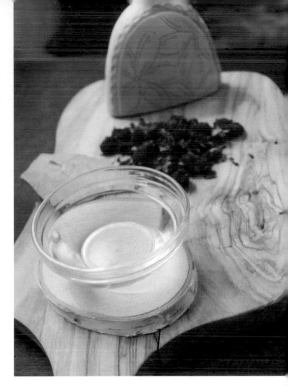

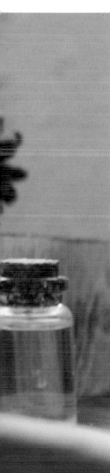

PART 6
Recipes for Face, Body, and Home 64

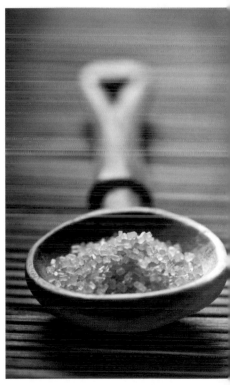

PART 1

Introduction

Finding healing in the plant kingdom is as old as time. There's an organic synergy between humans and plants; in fact, our very life—breath—depends on them. From ancient remedies to modern medicine, the plant world provides resources for healing. So, when essential oils began to be incorporated into more recent healing modalities, it was simply a continuation of the traditions of shamans, healers, and natural apothecaries. Only recently was the term "aromatherapy" coined, and like many things, it has come to be widely misunderstood as applying to anything that smells good—much of what currently passes for "aromatherapy" is full of chemically-created aromas that offer no aromatherapeutic benefits whatsoever. True healing benefits only come from the pure essential oils of plants.

THE SELF-CARE APOTHECARY

Building your home-care apothecary upon the foundation of essential oils creates a soothing, aromatically sensual system of self-care that is enjoyable, effective, and delightful to the senses.

The National Association for Holistic Aromatherapy (NAHA) describes the origins of the phrase "essential oil" as being

> a contraction of the original quintessential oil. This stems from the Aristotelian idea that matter is composed of four elements, namely, fire, air, earth, and water. The fifth element, or quintessence, was then considered to be spirit or life force.

Essential oils contain the concentrated *essence* of a plant, which includes chemical constituents that interact with human chemistry to alter mood and energy and provide medicinal benefits. They form the basis of the healing art of aromatherapy. This book integrates the benefits of aromatherapy with practical, daily-use products you can use to enhance your self-care routine.

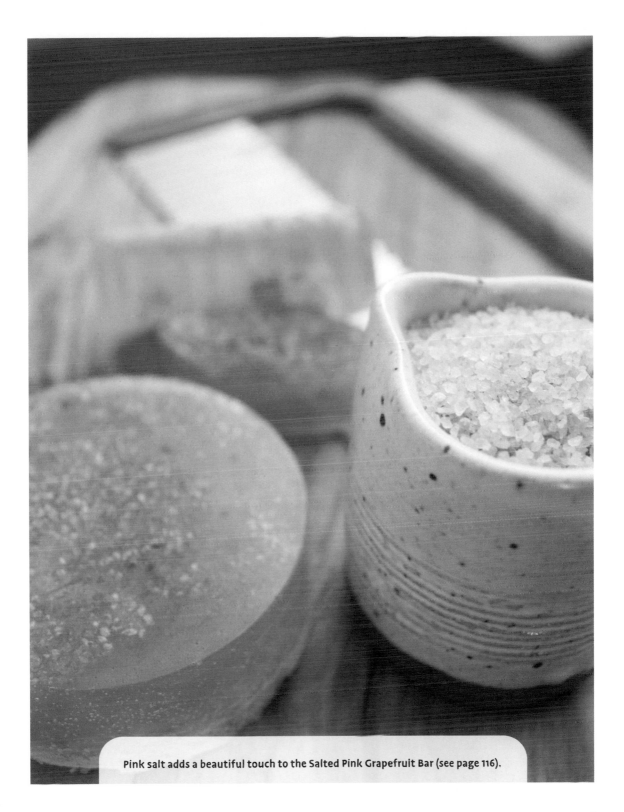

Pink salt adds a beautiful touch to the Salted Pink Grapefruit Bar (see page 116).

Investing in just a few essential oils and basic ingredients will allow you to fill your cupboards with your own luxurious creations—from cleansers and toothpastes to lotions and lip balms, all without adding any chemical scents. Instead, you'll create your bounty of botanical treasures with only pure essential oils—mixing homemade remedies to naturally boost your health, energy, and wellness.

Discovering the Power of Essential Oils

I discovered the power of essential oils after one of the most difficult moments of my life—the sudden loss of my son's father. The grief was all-consuming and seemingly impervious to any attempts to self-soothe—all but one. Somehow a small blend of rose and white pine found its way to my nightstand and inhaling the scent from that bottle of pure bliss was the only way I could find peaceful slumber. I didn't yet know how or why, but this little botanical bottle was my savior, a blend I now call "Grief Relief" (see page 47).

For a couple years prior to this breakthrough, I'd been making my own skin- and body-care

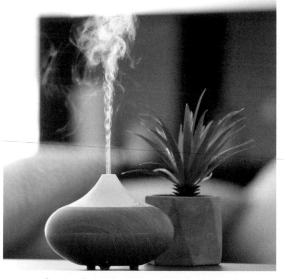

Scent and aroma have the power to evoke memories, soothe and comfort us, or energize us as we start our day.

products (soaps, lotions, and scrubs), but I'd been using synthetic fragrances and colors in my recipes. There's no denying that it can be fun to explore the variety of man-made options available—there's no natural way to bring mango, fig, or cucumber scents to your soaps, for example—but as I began to understand the benefits of pure essential oils, it started to feel disingenuous to use anything else in my products. After all, the point of making my own products was to bypass chemicals and create a greater sense of well-being. So, I made the decision that my creative space would be a 100 percent "chemical-free zone," relying entirely on the natural, healing aromas of essential oils. Several years later, I formalized my training with a 200-hour Professional Aromatherapy Certification course to gain a deeper understanding of the science behind essential oils.

The Art and Science of Aromatherapy

The term "aromatherapy" was first coined in 1937 by French perfumer and chemist René-Maurice Gattefossé, although humans have been using plant medicine since the beginning of time. The reason essential oils are so powerful is that our sense of smell was the first one to develop in mammals and it connects directly to the reptilian, or primal, brain. We react to scent emotionally because we're hardwired to. Aroma entices, excites, soothes, repels, comforts, evokes memories, and tickles the imagination.

Scent permeates some of our most enduring memories and acute experiences. It's why we remember pleasant, familiar smells from our childhood with such fondness, and why unpleasant smells can create such strong reactions. The aromas of fruits, flowers, resins, roots, barks, and seeds in the form of essential oils connect us to nature in a deep way. They literally bring nature into our homes—and our bodies—with all the same life-affirming benefits of a stroll through the forest.

ABOUT THE RECIPES

The recipes in this book are all plant-based and 100% natural except for the emulsifying wax and preservative necessary for lotions. I've avoided making shampoos and body washes, as those often require more synthetic ingredients. Where liquid washes are used, I've started with a 100 percent natural castile soap base—a wonderful starting place for customizing body and hair-care products with essential oils.

One thing to keep in mind is that natural ingredients can vary quite a bit by manufacturer, and your ratios may need tweaking. For example, the oat powder I purchase is very fine, so the oil quantity given for my Cherry Rose Face Scrub on page 78 is based on using that specific oat powder. Other brands sold may be coarser or more absorbent, requiring a slight increase in the quantity of oil you use. Always trust your judgment and adjust your quantities based on the behavior of your specific ingredients.

Just as with a cookbook, you'll know how much time and expense you want to invest! You can begin with just a few essential oils to make blends or pick a recipe or two that most appeal to you and purchase the necessary ingredients. The essential oil blends on pages 45–63, face mists on page 28, and lip balms on pages 104–107, for example, use very few ingredients and can easily get you started with three ingredients or less. As you start investing in more ingredients and tools, you'll soon find that your DIY products are more affordable and better for your skin and the environment than their big-box counterparts.

My intention is for you to both enjoy these recipes as is, but also see them as a jumping-off point for your own exploration and creativity. I've tried to keep the ingredient lists short and approachable, but there are so many wonderful botanicals to explore. I hope you'll be inspired to continue learning and creating your own natural products—it's a healing journey that will also free you from reliance on commercial brands and help you lower your carbon footprint.

WEIGHTS, MEASUREMENTS, AND CONVERSIONS

I'm in the U.S. and have used imperial measurements to make these recipes. Conversion to metric is included and, for difficult-to-measure ingredients (like very firm cocoa butter), I've measured by weight. Please keep in mind that variations in measuring techniques may create slight variations in the finished products. More conversions are easily found with an internet search, but the following chart will be helpful as you begin creating.

⅛ teaspoon = 0.5ml = 10 drops

¼ teaspoon = 1.25ml = 20 drops

1 teaspoon = 5ml = 100 drops

1 tablespoon = 15ml = 300 drops

1 ounce = 2 tablespoons = 6 teaspoons = 600 drops

1 pound = 16 ounces = 473ml = 0.47L

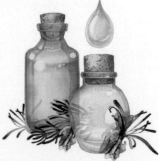

PART 2
About Essential Oils

Essential oils offer healing benefits because of their chemical profiles and the related effects on the human body. While we, of course, can enjoy their scent purely for pleasure, they also affect our health, healing, and happiness.

Eucalyptus stimulates the immune system and helps us breathe better. See page 18.

There are 10 types of essential oil chemical profiles, which have mood-soothing, antibacterial, pain-reducing, and other properties based on their chemical interaction with our physiology. Every essential oil has a predominant chemical family that drives its healing benefits. For example, lavender is an oil with a large quantity of esters, which help to regulate the nervous system, modulate immunity, and can be anti-inflammatory. And while each oil has a predominant chemical family, most include other chemical families as well, offering multidimensional, layered benefits.

ESSENTIAL OIL CHEMICAL FAMILIES

CHEMICAL FAMILY	OIL SOURCES	POPULAR OILS	BENEFITS
Monoterpenes	pines, spruces, firs, citruses	Lemon, Lime, Bergamot, Tangerine, Juniper, Nutmeg, Marjoram	antibacterial, antioxidant, balancing
Monoterpenols	leaves, flowers	Neroli, Rose, Geranium, Basil, Peppermint, Tea Tree, Lavender	antimicrobial, anti-inflammatory, antioxidant, calming, immune-supporting
Sesquiterpenes	woods, resins, roots	Cedar, Sandalwood, Myrrh, Vetiver, Balsam Copaiba, Patchouli, Spikenard, Ylang Ylang, German Chamomile, Black Pepper, Ginger	skin healing, anti-inflammatory, calming, soothing, antispasmodic.
Sesquiterpenols	woods, resins, roots, seeds	Sandalwood, Carrot Seed	skin healing, anti-inflammatory, calming, soothing, antispasmodic.
Ketones	seeds, bark, leaves	Rosemary, Buddha Wood, Sage, Peppermint, Wormwood	antiviral, analgesic, wound-healing
Oxides	leaves, seeds	Eucalyptus, Rosemary, Cardamom, Thyme	respiration-supporting, antiviral, anti-inflammatory
Esters	flowers, leaves	Jasmine, Roman Chamomile, Helichrysum, Lavender, Clary Sage, Petitgrain, Cardamom	skin-soothing, immunity-regulating
Ethers	seeds, leaves	Fennel, Tarragon, Parsley, Cardamom, Star Anise	antiparasitic, antifungal, digestion-supporting
Phenols	seeds, leaves	Clove, Cinnamon, Oregano, Thyme	antifungal, antimicrobial, antioxidant, toning, stimulating. *very strong and never to be used directly on the skin or near the eyes.*
Aldehydes	lemon-y sources	Lemon, Lemongrass, Citronella, Lemon Verbena, Lemon Myrtle, Melissa, May Chang	antifungal, antiviral, calming, bug-deterring, deodorizing

THE BENEFITS OF ESSENTIAL OILS

While all the recipes in this book can be made scent-free or with synthetic fragrances, the intention is to make use of the benefits of essential oils in each product. Essential oils exist in plants to provide antimicrobial properties, repel bugs, and prevent disease. When we realize we are biological beings related to plants on a molecular level, we can easily see why essential oils offer us similar benefits. The following are just a few of the areas in which essential oils can positively affect our lives.

Health and Wellness—Essential oils, such as peppermint, lemongrass, rosemary, and eucalyptus, can be antifungal, antibacterial, antiviral, immune-supporting, analgesic (pain-reducing), supportive of lung health, and fatigue-fighting. They contribute to our overall wellness, and integrating them into our skin, body, and home routines ensures seamless, consistent exposure to these healthful ingredients.

Mind and Mood—Essential oils have natural chemicals that affect our energy, inducing sleep and relaxation, promoting energy, or supporting positive moods. Lavender, frankincense, rose, and vetiver essential oils—among many others—can reduce anxiety, stress, insomnia, and depression, creating a feeling of optimism and a sense of balance.

Skin Health—Our skin often takes a beating, incurring burns, rashes, breakouts, and infections. Oils like chamomile, helichrysum, yarrow, clary sage, lavender, tea tree and frankincense soothe and support skin, offering natural remedies to these common maladies.

A CONCENTRATED POWER

Essential oils are a dramatically concentrated material. It takes 2,000 rose petals to create one drop of rose essential oil. A single drop of essential oil is equal to 40 cups of herbal tea and is 75 to 100 times more powerful than the fresh plant matter from which it's extracted.

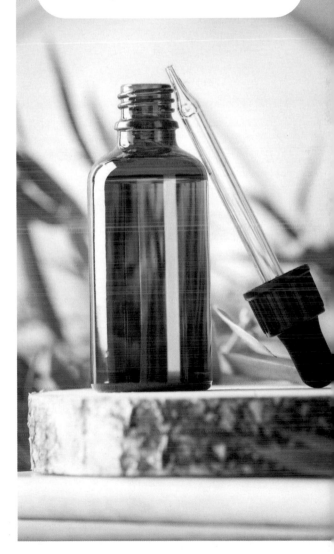

GETTING STARTED

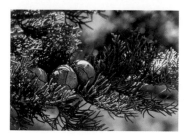

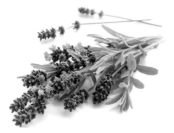

The Most *Essential* Essential Oils

I've included a larger list of many of the other essential oils used in my recipes (with a few more details about each) on pages 17-19, but if you want to begin creating within a more limited budget, you can use this "Top Ten" (included in alphabetical order) as a starter buying guide!

A balanced blend includes a top, middle, and base note, creating the most harmonious type of scent profile that will last longest on the skin.

CYPRESS

Harvested from the cones, leaves, twigs, and branches of *Cupressus sempervirens*
- Middle note
- Monoterpene family
- Mind-clearing, fresh, and foresty
- Analgesic, anti-inflammatory, antirheumatic, antispasmodic, decongestant
- Blends well with citrus-, floral-, and wood-based oils

LAVENDER

Harvested from the flower of *Lavandula angustifolia*
- Top/middle note
- Ester and Monoterpenol families
- Calming, soothing, floral, and herbaceous
- Mood-balancing, skin-healing, relaxing, anti-inflammatory
- Blends well with wood- and citrus-based oils

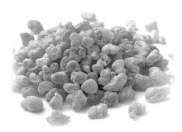

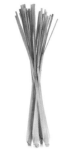

FRANKINCENSE

Harvested from the gum/resin of *Boswellia carterii*
- Base note
- Monoterpene family
- Invigorating, inspiring, light, soft, and woody
- Analgesic, antibacterial, and anti-inflammatory
- Blends well with floral- and resin-based oils

LEMONGRASS

Harvested from the grass of *Cymbopogon flexuosus*
- Middle/top note
- Aldehyde family
- Uplifting and bright
- Antianxiety, antidepressant, antifungal, antimicrobial
- Blends well with lavender, cedar, lime, and other citrus oils

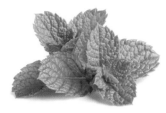

PEPPERMINT

Harvested from the leaves of
Mentha × piperita, a mint hybrid.

- Top/middle note
- Monoterpenol and
  Ketone families
- Energizing, cool, and fresh
- Analgesic, antidepressant,
  anti-inflammatory, antiseptic,
  decongestant, immune support
- Blends well with leaf- and
  citrus-based oils

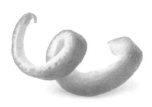

SWEET ORANGE

Harvested from the rind of
Citrus sinensus

- Top note
- Monoterpene family
- Mood-lifting, smooth,
  and sweet
- Antidepressant, antiviral,
  supports the liver
  and digestion
- Blends well with all oil types

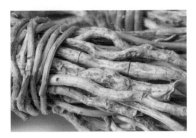

VETIVER

Harvested from the root of
Vetiveria zizanoides

- Base note
- Sesquiterpene, Sesquiterpenol,
  and Ketone families
- Grounding, earthy, and sweet
- Antidepressant, antifungal,
  antibacterial, deodorizing
- Blends well with floral-, citrus-,
  and wood-based oils

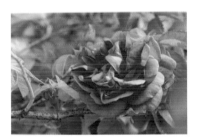

ROSE OTTO

Harvested from the flowers of
Rosa damascena

- Middle note
- Monoterpenol family
- Grounding, floral, and rich
- Antianxiety, antibacterial,
  antidepressant,
  antioxidant, aphrodisiac,
  calming, tonifying
- Blends well with wood- and
  seed-based oils

*Authentic rose essential oil is very
expensive, but worth every drop!*

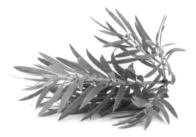

TEA TREE

Harvested from the leaves of
Melaleuca alternifolia

- Middle note
- Monoterpene and
  Monoterpenol families
- Herbaceous, fresh, and lemony
- Antibacterial, antifungal,
  antimicrobial, antiseptic,
  and antiviral
- Blends well with lavender,
  eucalyptus, lemon,
  and rosemary

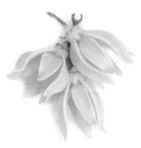

YLANG YLANG

Harvested from the flower of
Cananga odorata

- Middle/base note
- Sesquiterpene, Ester, and
  Monoterpenol families
- Uplifting, balancing, sensual,
  and sweet
- Analgesic, antianxiety,
  antidepressant, anti-
  inflammatory, antiseptic,
  aphrodisiac, and sedative
- Blends well with citrus- and
  wood-based oils

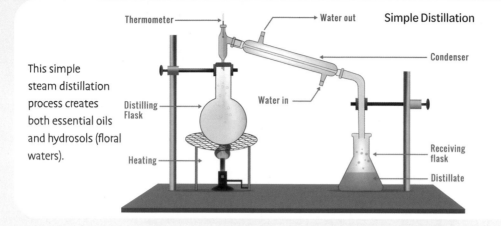

Thermometer — Water out — Simple Distillation

Condenser

Distilling Flask

Water in

Heating

Water out

Receiving flask

Distillate

This simple steam distillation process creates both essential oils and hydrosols (floral waters).

STEAM DISTILLATION

The most common method for producing essential oils is steam distillation. Plant matter is placed in a large container (a still) and steam is injected, causing the plant to release its oils in a vaporized state. They travel through a condenser, and two pipes separate the hot water, which exits, and the cold water, which enters the condenser. The vapor cools back into a liquid form within the condenser. Because water and oil do not mix, the essential oil can be siphoned from the water. The water left behind in this process is the hydrosol or "floral water."

CO$_2$ EXTRACTION

In CO$_2$ extraction, none of the constituents of the oil are damaged by heat, so it's higher quality and truer to the plant's original state. Instead of heated water or steam, CO$_2$ is used at temperatures between 95 to 100 degrees F (35 to 38 degrees C). Pressurized carbon dioxide acts as a solvent and is pumped into a chamber filled with plant matter, pulling the oils and other substances such as pigment and resin. The essential oil content then dissolves into the liquid CO$_2$. The CO$_2$ is brought back to natural

pressure and evaporates into its gaseous state, leaving the oil behind.

COLD PRESS EXTRACTION

In this process, used for citrus fruits like orange, lemon, grapefruit, and lime, the whole fruit is pressed to squeeze out both the juice and the oil. The liquid is then centrifuged to filter the solids and liquids. The oil separates from the juice and is captured.

MACERATION AND INFUSIONS

This is an easy, at-home way to create simple oils that have essential oil benefits. Crush and grind entirely dried-out plant matter (any moisture could create spoilage) into a coarse powder and add it to a carrier oil (see page 25). Add a solvent of your choosing and allow it to sit for a week, shaking occasionally. Strain and use the oil for massages or as a recipe ingredient.

ENFLEURAGE

A classic and largely outdated method is to press botanicals into animal or vegetable fat and let it sit for a few weeks to months, replacing the flowers daily, until the fat becomes

infused with the flower's fragrance compounds, creating an "enfleurage pomade." The pomade is washed with alcohol to separate the botanical extract from the remaining fat, which can then be used as an ingredient in soap or perfumery.

SOLVENT EXTRACTION

Food-grade solvents like hexane and ethanol are used to isolate essential oils from plant material. This process is usually used with sturdy plants (roots, resins, or woods) that yield low amounts of essential oil or delicate aromatics that are unable to withstand the pressure and distress of steam distillation. This method produces a finer fragrance than any type of distillation method, and is typically used in perfumery rather than aromatherapy, as the chemical solvents do not preserve the naturally healing benefits of the plant.

WATER DISTILLATION

Water distillation involves submerging fragile plant material in pure boiling water and allowing it to cool, whereby the oils and water separate into essential oil and hydrosol. This is mostly used for delicate flowers such as roses and orange blossoms.

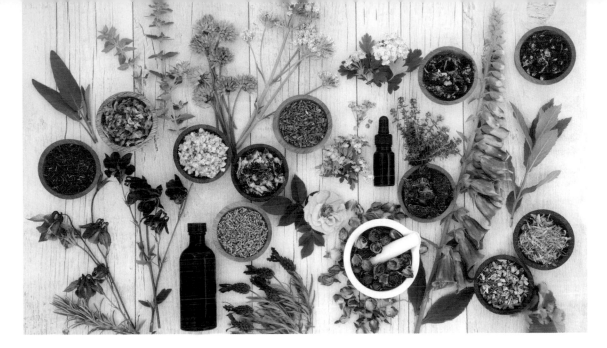

Recommended Essential Oils

There are hundreds of essential oils, and their scent profiles and benefits vary according to the unique soil, topography, and climate of the natural environment in which they are grown. One can spend a lifetime exploring and studying essential oils. Start small with Getting Started—The Most *Essential* Essential Oils on page 14 and use the following chart when you're ready to build a more comprehensive home apothecary.

OTHER ESSENTIAL OILS USED IN THIS BOOK

BERGAMOT
LATIN NAME: *Citrus bergamia*
PLANT PART: Peel
CHEMICAL PROFILE: Monoterpenes
BENEFITS: antianxiety, antibacterial, antidepressant, anti-inflammatory, antiviral, calming

BLACK SPRUCE
LATIN NAME: *Picea mariana*
PLANT PART: Needles
CHEMICAL PROFILE: Esters, Monoterpenes
BENEFITS: analgesic, anti-inflammatory, respiratory-therapeutic, antiseptic

CLOVE BUD
LATIN NAME: *Eugenia caryophyllata*
PLANT PART: Dried fruit
CHEMICAL PROFILE: Phenols
BENEFITS: antifungal, anti-inflammatory, antiviral, digestive stimulant, energizing, insect repellant, warming

BALSAM COPAIBA
LATIN NAME: *Copaifera officinalis*
PLANT PART: Gum/Resin
CHEMICAL PROFILE: Sesquiterpines
BENEFITS: anti-inflammatory, calming, wound-healing

CARDAMOM
LATIN NAME: *Elettaria cardamomum*
PLANT PART: Seed
CHEMICAL PROFILE: Esters, Oxides
BENEFITS: warming, anti-infectious, digestive stimulant

CEDARWOOD
LATIN NAME: *Juniperus virginiana*
PLANT PART: Wood
CHEMICAL PROFILE: Sesquiterpenes
BENEFITS: antifungal, anti-infectious, respiratory decongestant

OTHER ESSENTIAL OILS USED IN THIS BOOK

CHAMOMILE, ROMAN
LATIN NAME: *Anthemis nobilis*
PLANT PART: Flower
CHEMICAL PROFILE: Esters
BENEFITS: pain relief, promotes sense of well-being, skin-soothing

CITRONELLA
LATIN NAME: *Cymbopogon winterianus*
PLANT PART: Grass
CHEMICAL PROFILE: Aldehydes, Monoterpenes, Monoterpenols
BENEFITS: insect repellant, analgesic, antibacterial, antifungal, deodorizing

CLARY SAGE
LATIN NAME: *Salvia sclarea*
PLANT PART: Leaf/Flower Bud
CHEMICAL PROFILE: Esters
BENEFITS: skin-soothing, mood-boosting, hormone-regulating

EUCALYPTUS
LATIN NAME: *Eucalyptus globulus*
PLANT PART: Leaves
CHEMICAL PROFILE: Oxides
BENEFITS: anti-infectious, antiviral, decongestant, immune-supporting

GERANIUM ROSE
LATIN NAME: *Pelargonium graveolens*
PLANT PART: Leaves
CHEMICAL PROFILE: Monoterpenols, Esters
BENEFITS: mood-balancing, skin-soothing, anti-inflammatory

GINGER
LATIN NAME: *Zingiber officinale*
PLANT PART: Root
CHEMICAL PROFILE: Sesquiterpenes, Monoterpenes
BENEFITS: analgesic, warming, antiviral, antibacterial, anti-inflammatory, antioxidant, antimicrobial, supports digestion

GRAPEFRUIT, PINK
LATIN NAME: *Citrus paradisii*
PLANT PART: Rind
CHEMICAL PROFILE: Monoterpenes
BENEFITS: analgesic, antianxiety, antidepressant, anti-inflammatory, antioxidant, immune-supporting

HELICHRYSUM
LATIN NAME: *Helichrysum italicum*
PLANT PART: Flowers
CHEMICAL PROFILE: Esters, Monoterpenes, Sesquiterpenes
BENEFITS: skin-soothing, anti-allergenic, anti-inflammatory, analgesic, wound-healing

JASMINE
LATIN NAME: *Jasminum grandiflorum*
PLANT PART: Flower
CHEMICAL PROFILE: Esters, Monoterpenols
BENEFITS: uplifting, antidepressant, skin-soothing

JUNIPER BERRY
LATIN NAME: *Juniperus communis*
PLANT PART: Berries
CHEMICAL PROFILE: Monoterpenes
BENEFITS: antirheumatic, stimulant, tonic

LEMON
LATIN NAME: *Citrus limon*
PLANT PART: Rind
CHEMICAL PROFILE: Monoterpenes
BENEFITS: antimicrobial, antibacterial, uplifting

LEMON EUCALYPTUS
LATIN NAME: *Eucalyptus citriodora*
PLANT PART: Leaves
CHEMICAL PROFILE: Aldehydes
BENEFITS: bug repellant, antibacterial, antifungal, antiseptic

LEMON MYRTLE
LATIN NAME: *Backhousia citriodora*
PLANT PART: Leaves
CHEMICAL PROFILE: Aldehydes
BENEFITS: antianxiety, antidepressant, antiviral, calming, sedative, disinfectant

LEMON VERBENA
LATIN NAME: *Lippia citriodora*
PLANT PART: Leaves
CHEMICAL PROFILE: Aldehydes, Monoterpenes
BENEFITS: calming, analgesic, antibacterial, antidepressant, antifungal, anti-inflammatory, antimicrobial, antioxidant

OTHER ESSENTIAL OILS USED IN THIS BOOK

LIME
LATIN NAME: *Citrus aurantifolia*
PLANT PART: Rind
CHEMICAL PROFILE: Monoterpenes
BENEFITS: antianxiety, antibacterial, antidepressant, anti-infectious, antioxidant, antiviral, decongestant, tonic

MANDARIN, RED
LATIN NAME: *Citrus reticulata var mandarin*
PLANT PART: Rind
CHEMICAL PROFILE: Monoterpenes
BENEFITS: analgesic, antianxiety, antibacterial, antidepressant, anti-inflammatory, antioxidant, antiviral, digestive tonic, carminative, expectorant

MARJORAM, SWEET
LATIN NAME: *Origanum majorana*
PLANT PART: Leaves
CHEMICAL PROFILE: Monoterpenes, Monoterpenols
BENEFITS: antibacterial, antifungal, anti-inflammatory, antimicrobial, antioxidant, antiviral, calming, immune stimulant

MENTHOL
LATIN NAME: *Mentha arvensis*
PLANT PART: Leaves
CHEMICAL PROFILE: Monoterpenes
BENEFITS: soothing, cooling, stimulating, analgesic

MYRRH
LATIN NAME: *Commiphora myrrha*
PLANT PART: Gum/Resin
CHEMICAL PROFILE: Sesquiterpenes
BENEFITS: respiratory decongestant, skin-soothing, anti-inflammatory, antibacterial, antimicrobial, analgesic, expectorant, mucolytic, astringent, calming, wound-healing

NEROLI
LATIN NAME: *Citrus aurantium var amara*
PLANT PART: Flowers
CHEMICAL PROFILE: Monoterpenes, Monoterpenols, Esters, Sesquiterpenols
BENEFITS: antidepressant, soothing, analgesic, antianxiety, immune-supporting, sedative, tonic, aphrodisiac

PINE, SCOTCH
LATIN NAME: *Pinus sylvestris*
PLANT PART: Needles
CHEMICAL PROFILE: Monoterpenes
BENEFITS: analgesic, decongestant, anti-inflammatory, antioxidant

ROSEMARY
LATIN NAME: *Salvia rosmarinus ct cineole*
PLANT PART: Leaves
CHEMICAL PROFILE: Oxides, Monoterpenes, Ketones
BENEFITS: analgesic, antibacterial, antioxidant, digestive tonic, respiratory-supporting

THYME
LATIN NAME: *Thymus vulgaris*
PLANT PART: Flowers, Leaves
CHEMICAL PROFILE: Monoterpenes, Phenols
BENEFITS: antimicrobial, antifungal, antiviral, analgesic, antioxidant, immune-supporting

SAGE, WHITE
LATIN NAME: *Salvia apiana*
PLANT PART: Leaves
CHEMICAL PROFILE: Oxides
BENEFITS: antibacterial, antimicrobial, antiseptic, antiviral, decongestant, energizing

SANDALWOOD
LATIN NAME: *Santalum spicatum*
PLANT PART: Wood
CHEMICAL PROFILE: Sesquiterpenols
BENEFITS: analgesic, antianxiety, antifungal, anti-inflammatory, antiseptic, sedative

YARROW
LATIN NAME: *Achillea millefolium*
PLANT PART: Flowers, Leaves
CHEMICAL PROFILE: Monoterpenes, Sesquiterpenes
BENEFITS: analgesic, anti-inflammatory, antioxidant, antiviral, calming, digestive tonic, immune-supporting

YUZU
LATIN NAME: *Citrus junos*
PLANT PART: Rind
CHEMICAL PROFILE: Monoterpenes
BENEFITS: antibacterial, antidepressant, antiseptic, antiviral, carminative, sedative

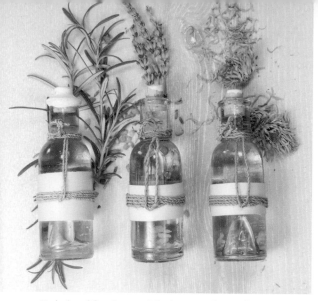

Herbal and floral essential oils mix well together to create soothing, energizing blends.

SOURCING YOUR ESSENTIAL OILS

Unfortunately, fraudulent essential oils are readily available online. Some of the oils you find available via big-box online retailers sell for only $10, while a true essential oil from the plant in question would be 20 times that price. These are fake imports from overseas. Don't be deceived, as they will not deliver the therapeutic benefits you're working toward. It's better to purchase from a reputable essential oil distributor and pay the true cost for a very small amount, since you only need a few drops for each blend. Credible essential oil sellers will make available a Gas Chromatography Mass Spectrometry (GC/MS) report for each oil, listing its chemical profile and verifying that the batch has been tested and is authentic.

ESSENTIAL OIL STORAGE AND SAFETY

Essential oils are volatile and best kept in dark bottles in a cool place to avoid premature rancidity. When kept properly, oils will last many months or even years. Some of the lighter, "top note" oils, like those extracted from citrus fruits, remain potent for one to two years, while deeper oils extracted from resins and roots can last many years without degradation. I've taken to keeping citrus oils in the refrigerator to ensure the longest life possible.

Don't put oils directly on your skin ("neat" application). Instead, use them in a carrier oil. Sensitivities are personal, and if an oil causes redness or discomfort of any kind, discontinue use immediately. The quickest way to soothe a bad reaction is to immediately apply a mild carrier oil, such as olive or sunflower oil to dilute its affect on your skin. Never ingest essential oils.

If you are pregnant or nursing, avoid anise, ho leaf, carrot seed, cassia/cinnamon, cypress, and fennel. Many other oils may be prohibited, especially those in these chemical families: ketones, phenols, oxides, ethers, esters, and aldehydes. Be sure to research which oils to avoid entirely and consult with a professional before using any oils while pregnant or nursing.

There is a phenomenon called phototoxicity whereby certain oils containing molecules called furanocoumarins (FCs) can cause skin to be sensitive to the sun. Avoid use of the following essential oils before sun exposure: cold-pressed bergamot, lime, lemon, grapefruit, other citruses, cumin, and angelica root. **Note:** if these same plants are steam distilled, the essential oil is not phototoxic.

To learn the composition of any oil, refer to its GC/MS report—the "fingerprint" of a specific batch of oil that outlines its chemical composition. Reputable essential oil vendors will always provide these reports. For a comprehensive list of phototoxic oils and others not recommended for pregnancy, as well as extensive information on essential oil safety, I recommend referring to *Essential Oil Safety* by Robert Tisserand and Rodney Young.

20 QUICK WAYS TO INCORPORATE ESSENTIAL OILS INTO YOUR LIFE

1.
Carry a mist in your purse to refresh and restore your mood and energy any time you need it.

2.
Carry a small bottle of diluted oil in your yoga or gym bag and dab it on your wrists before beginning your workout.

3.
When traveling, have a face mist ready to wake up tired skin and give yourself an energy boost.

4.
Massage your hands, ears, and feet each morning with oil blends or essential oil creams to stimulate your lymphatic system.

5.
At bedtime, dab Sleep Support oil (see page 46) under your eyes and nose and massage it into the backs of your hands to help you sleep peacefully.

6.
Enhance cuddle time with your canine or feline friend by rubbing 2 drops of a floral or citrus oil between your palms and then petting them for 5–10 minutes. This bonding time can lower your blood pressure and provide a tremendous sense of wellbeing.

7.
Another pet bonding practice is to shake some dry shampoo (see page 124) into your dog's brush and slowly brush their coat until it's distributed. They will love it!

8.
Before sitting for meditation, dab a drop under your nose to inhale throughout your session.

9.
Add a few drops to a diffuser. Diffusers are great in bathrooms, bedrooms, and entranceways.

10.
Do yoga near a diffuser, inhaling deeply.

11.
Hang a car diffuser clip in your car to distribute essential oils while on the go.

12.
Add 5–6 drops to a couple tablespoons of a carrier oil mixed with a bit of sea salt. Add to a hot bath and soak.

13.
Mist your pillow before napping or sleeping.

14.
Keep a mist in your shower. Spritz and breathe deeply whenever you turn it on.

15.
On a cold winter day, add several drops of oil to the log on top before lighting your fire.

16.
When congested, add 2 drops of eucalyptus or rosemary oil to steaming water. Cover your head with a towel and breathe in the steam for 2–3 minutes.

17.
Add a couple drops of oil to your candles before lighting them.

18.
Add a drop or two to neti pot salts, then shake and allow the mixture to sit overnight and infuse. Use the salts as normal.

19.
Wear an essential oil diffuser necklace or bracelet for instant access to aromatherapy any time.

20.
Drop your favorite oils onto a cotton swab and carry it in your purse to use as a "sniffing stick" when needed. (The fastest way to benefit from essential oils is through inhalation!)

PART 3
Other Ingredients

This book covers an array of home-based products, from soaps and lotions to scrubs and cleaners, for a total home apothecary based on natural botanicals. In addition to essential oils, the ingredients in this section will allow you to make all the products in this book. **Note:** Since a percentage of what goes on your body goes in your body, I recommend buying organic whenever you can.

100% PLANT-BASED

For the health of the planet and our animal friends, all ingredients used in these recipes are plant-based. When purchasing ingredients, check with the manufacturer to confirm that their options are cruelty-free.

There are many important elements to creating spa-worthy products at home. Mixing in whole ingredients sometimes adds that special touch.

A REMINDER—USING NATURAL PRODUCTS

Unlike commercial brands, which tend to use the same vendors and ingredients, natural products vary depending on the source of your raw ingredients. I've had oat powders that are substantially different in texture and performance, depending on the vendor from whom I purchased them. Essential oils can also vary in aroma and potency based on the growing conditions and country of origin of the source plant. I recommend finding a vendor you trust and purchasing from them exclusively so you can create consistent products.

Even clays, powders, butters, and carrier oils can vary depending on where they are sourced and how they are processed. Remember to adjust the recipes in this book as needed based on your ingredients and desired results. My recipes were developed with the ingredients I have and may need tweaking if your ingredients are different in texture, consistency, or aroma.

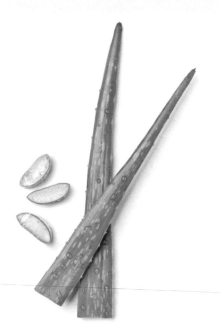

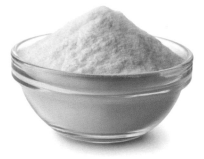

Baking Soda—Sodium bicarbonate ground to a fine powder is gently abrasive and dissolves dirt and grease. *Used in cleaning products and toothpaste.*

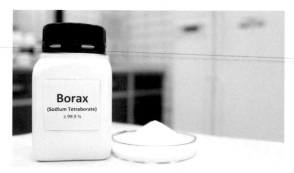

Aloe Vera—The inner gel of the aloe vera leaf, available as aloe vera water (juice) or aloe vera gel, is healing and soothing to skin. Aloe vera can get moldy quickly, so commercial-grade aloe vera is always sold with a preservative and may also include a thickener, like agar, to make a gel. Leave aloe vera in the refrigerator and use it with a preservative in any water-based products. *Used in lotions, masks, and toners.*

Borax—Sodium borate, the hydrate salt of boric acid, is an inhibitor of fungi and mold that absorbs dirt when used in skin and cleaning products. *Used in cleaning products.*

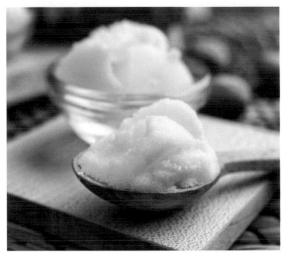

Butters Extracted from the pits and seeds of mango, shea, cocoa, pistachio, and other fruits, butters are full of fatty acids and nutrients that are wonderful for the skin. They each have their own textures and qualities—cocoa butter is much harder than mango butter, for example—but, for the most part, they can be used interchangeably in recipes. The final texture and weight will be affected by the butter you choose, however. *Used in lotions, balms, and butters.*

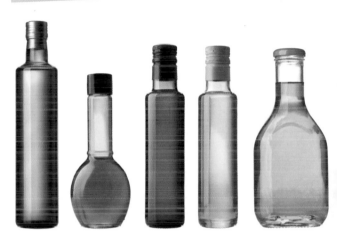

Carrier Oils—Plant oils compressed from seeds and nuts, such as avocado, coconut, almond, olive, apricot kernel, pomegranate, cherry kernel, grapeseed, and sunflower oil, that are used as dispersants for essential oils and other ingredients. They offer hydration and vitamins and nutrients to the skin with minimal to no aroma. Feel free to substitute the oils you have on hand in any recipe. *Used in lotions, scrubs, masks, and blends.*

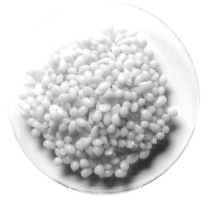

Candelilla Wax—A plant-based alternative to beeswax extracted from the candelilla plant, a desert shrub. *Used in balms and salves.*

Castile Soap—A natural, biodegradable, liquid soap typically made from olive, avocado, coconut, hemp, or other vegetable oils. Castile soap acts as a naturally cleansing base that can be customized with essential oils. *Used in face and body washes.*

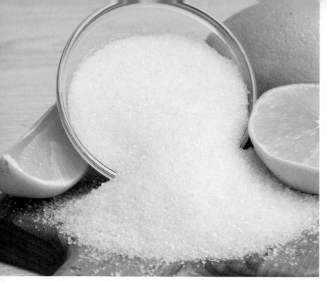

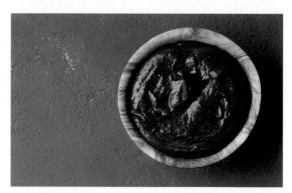

Dead Sea Mud—A mud extracted from the Dead Sea that has a high mineral and salt content. Dead Sea mud is clarifying, healing, and antimicrobial. *Used in masks and infused soap bars.*

Citric Acid—An acid extracted from citrus fruit that acts as a pH adjustor, protective antioxidant, exfoliator, and thickening agent. *Used in lotions.*

Cleaning Vinegar—An acidic liquid produced through fermentation (cleaning vinegar is 6 percent acid, higher than other kinds), which removes grease, dirt, and debris from surfaces. *Used in cleaning products.*

Distilled Water—Demineralized water that's been heated until it turns to vapor and then condensed back into water, leaving behind mineral residues. The resulting purified liquid creates a clean base for any water-based products. *Used in lotions.*

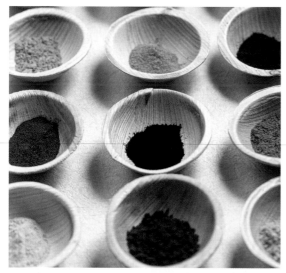

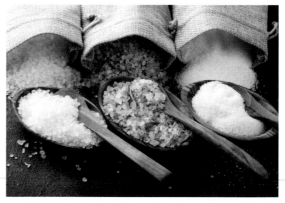

Colorants—Natural colorants such as spirulina, turmeric, coffee, and beetroot powder. They also act as gentle exfoliants in some products. *Used in soaps and scrubs.*

Exfoliants—Textured ingredients meant to slough off the top layer of dead skin to reveal radiant, clear skin. Could be clays, oat powder, rose petal powder, powdered apricot kernels and cherry seeds, dried blueberry and cranberry seeds, orange peel powder, rice husk powder, powdered walnuts, ground coffee, salts, sugars (white, brown, or coconut), sand, powdered coconut shell, etc. In general, use finer grains like powders for facial scrubs and larger grains like salt and sugar for body scrubs. *Used in scrubs.*

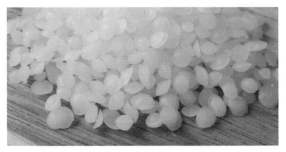

Emulsifying Wax (E-Wax)—A commercial wax product made from plant-based fatty acids that is used to emulsify water and oil in lotions and creams. Natural waxes cannot be substituted for this wax, which is specially formulated and essential to creating a lotion that won't separate. *Used in lotions and creams.*

Germaben® II—Germaben II is a necessary preservative for any water- or food-based products like lotions, creams, products with oat powder, or aloe-based products. It contains propylene glycol, propylparaben, methylparaben, and diazolidinyl urea and inhibits microbial, yeast, and mold growth. *Used in lotions and creams.*

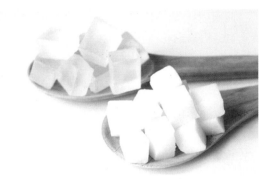

Glycerin Soap Blocks—Premade soap blocks that are clear if created with olive or coconut oil or opaque and white if made with shea butter. You can use them for the "melt and pour" process, in which you cut the blocks, melt them, infuse the liquid with your own botanicals and essential oils, and pour it into molds to create a customized soap bar. *Used in soap bars.*

Glycerin Liquid—Liquid typically made from soybean, coconut, or palm oil that acts as a humectant: it helps hydrate and seal in ingredients and also softens skin. Be sure to use plant-based glycerin. *Used in lotions and scrubs.*

Grapefruit Seed Extract (GSE)—An extract from grapefruit seeds that provides antioxidant benefits to the skin and acts as a natural microbial agent with some preservative qualities. *Used in lotions, balms, and scrubs.*

A NOTE ON OTHER SCENTS AND OILS

There are many scents that are delightful and pleasurable but aren't essential oils. For example, there are vanilla extracts, infusions, absolutes, and fragrance oils, but there's no true pure vanilla essential oil. Other scents we commonly see used in products are fig, cucumber, strawberry, mango, and coconut—all of which come from synthetic fragrance oils. There are strawberry and cucumber oils made from their pressed seeds (like olive and avocado oils), but, while they work well as carrier oils, they are not essential oils and don't offer any aromatherapeutic benefits.

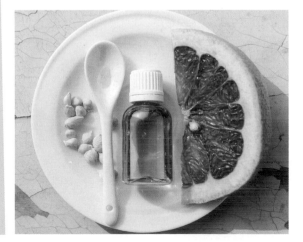

PURE HYDROSOL FACE MIST VARIATIONS

One of the beautiful byproducts of essential oil production is hydrosol—the water left behind when the steam distillation process separates the oil from the water. This water retains the chemical benefits of the plant, with all its healing qualities. Hydrosols are also referred to as floral waters.

Use any floral water on its own as a pure and natural way to tone and refresh your face. Simply pour it into a mister bottle and spritz it on your face after cleansing or at any time for light hydration and to refresh and wake up your skin or use it with a cotton pad after cleansing to tone and remove traces of dirt. **NOTE:** Unless a preservative is added, floral waters are best kept refrigerated when not in use.

FOR OILY SKIN, try geranium, rosemary, tea tree, frankincense, clary sage, lemon, or neroli hydrosol.

FOR DRY SKIN, try lavender, chamomile, sandalwood, myrrh, or patchouli hydrosol.

Hydrosol/Floral Water—The gentler, water-based byproduct of essential oil distillation. When plant matter is steam distilled, the steam reconstitutes in the form of water, retaining many of the same properties as the essential oil. Hydrosols have a soft, subtle scent. Unlike essential oils, hydrosols can be safely used directly on your skin and are wonderful for creating facial products. *Used in face and room mists.*

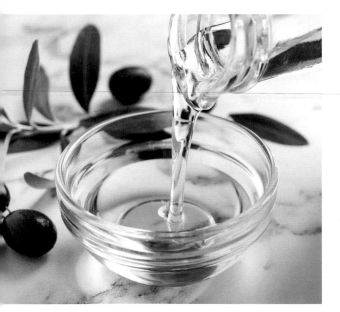

A LONG TRADITION—JOJOBA

Jojoba is native to the southwestern United States, and American Indians first made use of its treasures. After softening jojoba seeds with heat, they used a mortar and pestle to create a salve or buttery substance, which was then applied to the skin and hair to heal and condition.

Jojoba—A liquid form of plant wax extracted from jojoba seeds that won't clog pores. Jojoba helps treat acne, eczema, and other skin problems. It's similar to our own skin's sebum and is a wonderful addition to any lotion or face scrub. *Used in lotions, balms, butters, and scrubs.*

Orange Wax—Wax extracted from orange peels acts as a plant-based lanolin alternative to provide emollient and antioxidant benefits to the skin. It has an intense orange color and aroma. *Used in cleaning and hair styling products.*

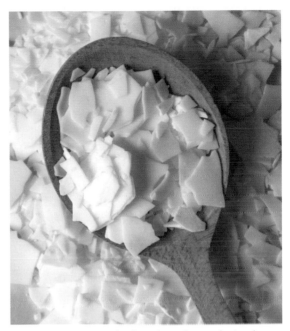

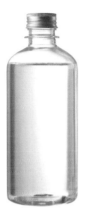

Perfumer's Alcohol—A formulation containing ethanol, isopropyl myristate, and monopropylene glycol that allows for smooth dispersion of essential oils without adding an overtly alcoholic aroma. It also preserves the essential oils to create a long-lasting room, face, or body mist that remains clear and well-mixed. *Used for mists and room sprays.*

Pumice Stone Powder—Pumice powder for crafting is made from volcanic ash and is used to add exfoliation to soap products. It is available from soap ingredient suppliers. *Used in soap bars.*

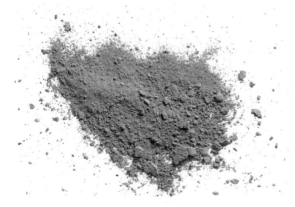

Soy Wax—A natural, plant-based wax derived from soybeans that works well in candles. It's a cruelty-free alternative to beeswax. *Used in candles.*

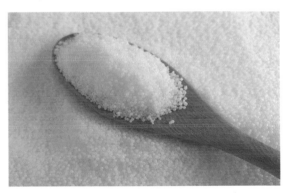

Stearic Acid—Hydrolyzed fat from animal or plant sources that thickens, texturizes, and stabilizes emulsions while lubricating and softening the skin. Confirm with manufacturer that their stearic acid is plant-based. *Used in lotions.*

Witch Hazel—A distillation from the leaves, bark, and twigs of the witch hazel plant that soothes and reduces inflammation, fights bacteria, and tones and tightens the skin. *Used in toners and aftershaves.*

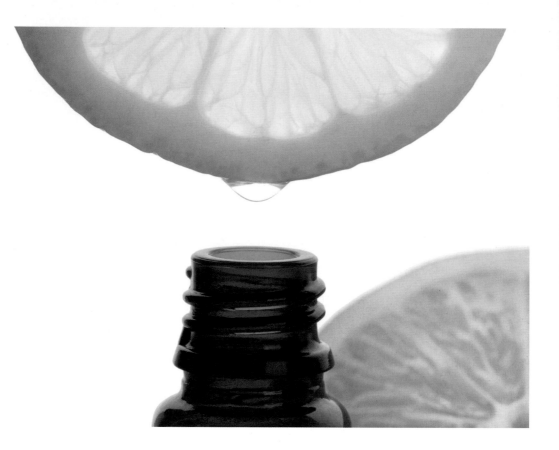

SHELF LIFE

While natural products in general are best when used frequently, when made properly (and with preservatives where necessary) they can have a shelf life of many years. I have creams I made at least five years ago that still maintain their consistency and fragrance without degradation! I can say the same for aromatherapy blends, soaps, and cleansers. In general, anything with aloe vera, oat powder, or a water- or food-based ingredient will need to be used within a few weeks or refrigerated.

Without chemical stabilizers, scrubs and masks can dry out over time—simply add a bit more of your favorite carrier oil and stir to rehydrate them. If you choose not to use a preservative in water-based products, keep them in the refrigerator to avoid the potential for mold. If humidity is a concern where you live, use a preservative!

If lotions separate, which doesn't typically happen because of the use of e-wax, simply shake or stir them. For water-based products, always shake them before use to reincorporate the ingredients. Keep them out of extremely hot environments, like hot cars, as this will change the consistency and could cause rancidity. With that being said, in 20 years of making and using these products, I've very rarely seen mold. In my experience, most products last for months and even years without any degradation in quality. Once made, they are quite shelf-stable when used regularly or kept refrigerated as necessary.

NATURAL PRODUCT SHELF LIFE—QUICK REFERENCE

PRODUCT	ESTIMATED SHELF LIFE
Balms, salves, butters, and creams	Years. No need for refrigeration, just avoid excessive heat (cars, etc.)
Salts, scrubs, and massage oils	Years, without refrigeration. If your scrub includes aloe vera or oat powder, keep refrigerated or add a preservative. Scrubs will dry out over time but can be restored easily with more carrier oil.
Soap—solid or liquid	Years
Aromatherapy blends—oil or mist	Years, when used in a carrier oil or with perfumer's alcohol. If you use another dispersant (like floral water), keep refrigerated or use within a few weeks. Depending on the essential oils used, the scent will fade over time but they are not prone to mold or rancidity.
Deodorant, spray cleansers, and powdered detergents	Years, without refrigeration or preservatives. Powders can dry out over time.
Face mists (aloe-based) and food-based face masks or scrubs (avocado, mango, or oat powder)	Keep refrigerated and use within a few days.

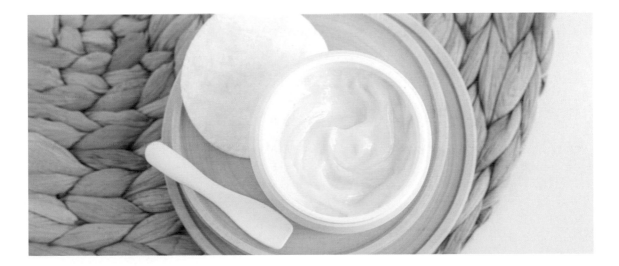

PART 4

Equipment

With a few tools and basic equipment, you can make all the recipes in this book. Most you'll already have in your kitchen.

Making home and body products is similar to cooking—and you use a lot of the same tools.

The basic kitchen equipment listed on these pages (mixing bowls, a smoothie blender, measuring cups and spoons, a kitchen scale, etc.) will work for creating all of the essential oil recipes in the book. There are other optional items listed that will make your creative process and the related cleanup just a little bit easier (wax paper is a nice option for turning out cut soap bars, for example, but a plate or cutting board works just as well).

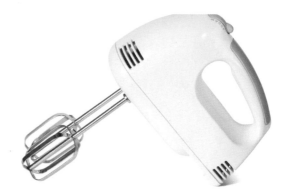

Electric Mixer—An electric mixer makes whipping up body butter a breeze. *Used for body butter.*

Essential Oil Bottle Opener—To remove the plastic nozzle in an essential oil bottle and allow for dropper insertion. *Used for all recipes as needed.*

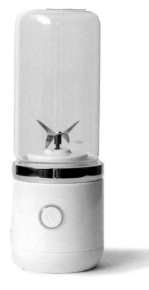

Blender (small, smoothie-style)—To easily mix ingredients for lotion and infused soap bars. *Used for lotions, creams, and soap bars.*

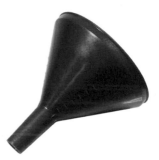

Funnel—Use to neatly pour ingredients and finished products into containers. *Used for lip balm, aromatherapy blends, lotions, and cleaners.*

Glass Measuring Cup—Pyrex® or similar glass measuring cups are the most convenient vessel for heating up ingredients for balms and lotions, as you can then pour the finished product directly into containers. *Used for lotions, balms, and infused soaps.*

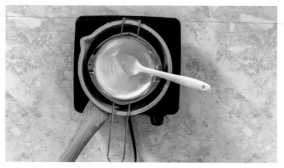

Double Boiler—Used to safely melt wax and oils to a pourable consistency. *Used for balms, butters, salves, and candles.*

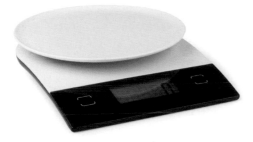

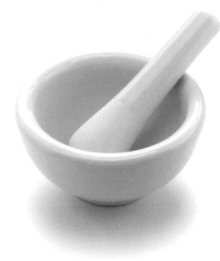

Kitchen Scale—A kitchen scale will let you precisely measure your ingredients, making sure your final product has exactly the texture and scent you were working to achieve. *Used for all recipes as needed.*

Mortar and Pestle or Coffee Grinder—Used to prepare dried herbs and flowers and to create powders. *Used for soaps and scrubs.*

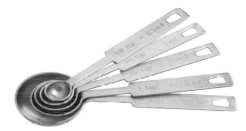

Measuring Spoons—These are indispensable tools for accurately measuring ingredients. *Used for scrubs, lotions, creams, cleansers, soaps, blends, and candles.*

Paper Towels—For easy cleanup of spills and overflow. Since these recipes include oils and waxes that are not easily washed, I don't recommend using cloth towels. Use reusable bamboo and recycled paper towels to be a bit greener! *Used for all recipes as needed.*

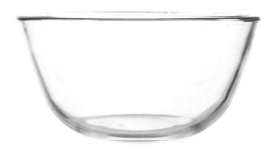

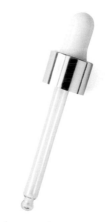

Mixing Bowls—You'll need a mixing bowl or two that is easy to clean and won't absorb essential oils. Glass is the best option, but bamboo, aluminum, and ceramic bowls work, as well. *Used for soaps, scrubs, toothpaste, and butters.*

Pipettes—Glass or plastic pipettes used to draw and disperse essential oils into blends and recipes. *Used for most recipes as needed.*

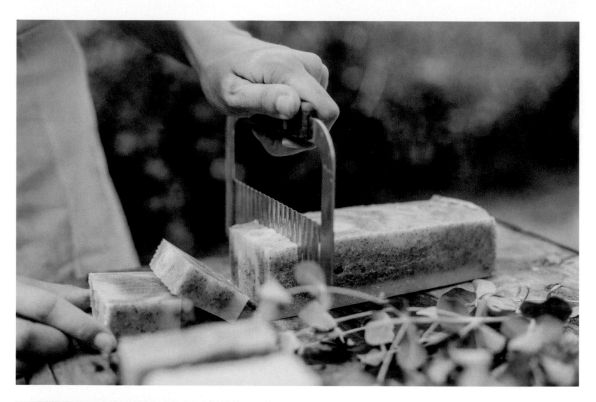

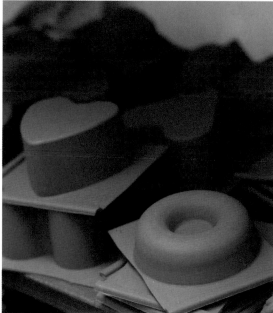

Soap Cutter—Special straight or curved-edge cutters with handles for convenient soap block cutting. You can also use a large kitchen knife if you don't want to purchase a separate soap cutter. *Used for soaps made with a block mold rather than a shaped mold.*

Soap Mold—To pour melted soap into. Soap molds are available in block or fun, shaped forms. The recipes in this book use 4-ounce shaped molds, but you can also use a block mold and cut your soap to size. *Used for infused soaps.*

Stirring Spoons (silicone, bamboo, or wood)—Dedicate a few select spoons for stirring your creations. *Used for soaps, scrubs, toothpaste, and butters.*

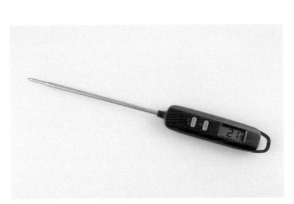

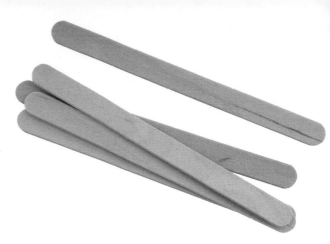

Thermometer—Test the temperature of water and oil before blending until you get more experience with the materials. *Used for lotions.*

Wooden Craft Sticks or Clothespins—Place these across the top of your candle containers to hold your wicks upright as the wax dries. *Used for candles.*

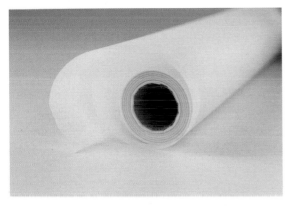

Wax Paper—Used for turning out soap bars. You can also use a plate or cutting board if you don't have wax paper available. *Used for soap bars.*

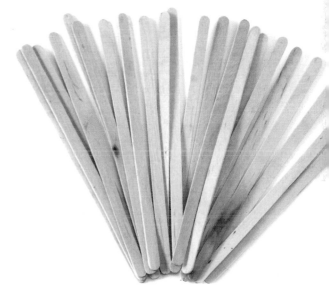

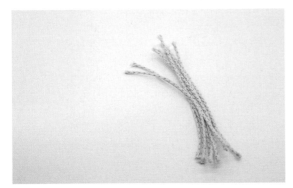

Wooden Stir Sticks—Instead of spoons, use disposable wooden stir sticks when only a small quantity needs to be mixed. These make for easier cleanup. *Used for scrubs, soaps, balms, and toothpaste.*

Wicks with Adhesive—Apply these to the bottom inside of your candle containers before you pour in wax. *Used for candles.*

CLEANING YOUR TOOLS

In general, the sooner you clean your equipment the easier it will be. Once you've packaged your products, most of the tools can be immediately submerged in hot, soapy water for easy cleaning. Mixing bowls, blenders, stirring spoons, and measuring spoons and cups can all go directly into hot soapy water to be washed out before they dry.

If you do find yourself with dried wax in a glass bowl or measuring cup, simply add some water and microwave it for about a minute until it's hot, then pour out the water and wipe out the wax with a paper towel. For dried wax on metal, you can submerge the tool in very hot water to soften the wax, then use paper towels to scrape it off.

I like to use glass pipettes for dropping in essential oils, but plastic pipettes are still washable and reusable many times over. When I'm blending, I keep a small bowl with rubbing alcohol nearby so once I've finished using a pipette (whether glass or plastic), I can draw in the alcohol a few times, expel it, and then place the cleaned pipette on a towel or in a cup to dry.

PACKAGING OPTIONS

For packaging your creations, keep an assortment of tins, small and large glass jars, small spray bottles, paper tubes of various sizes, and 8-ounce (250ml) glass bottles (for body oils, bath salts, and face washes) on hand. You can also repurpose glass food jars by running them through the dishwasher first to disinfect them and peel the labels off. For cleaning sprays, I buy 16-ounce (500ml) glass spray bottles, but for my laundry detergents and dishwashing soaps, I repurpose little buckets, pails, and jars I find around the house—part of the fun of making DIY products is getting creative with your packaging.

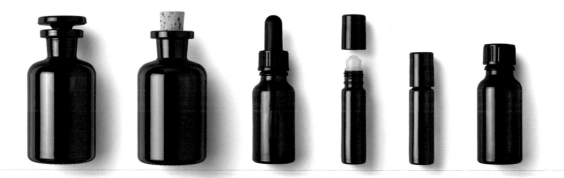

Dropper and Roller Ball Bottles (5ml, 10ml, 15ml, 30ml)—Used to package skin-based aromatherapy blends.

Glass Jars with Lids (2-ounce, 4-ounce, 8-ounce)—Used to package lotions, cremes, scrubs, butters, toothpaste, deodorant, masks, and cleansers.

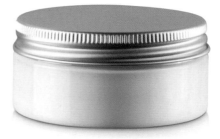

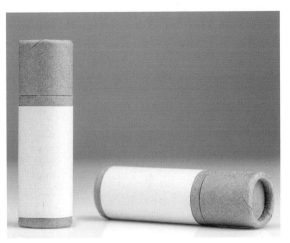

Paper Tubes (small, medium)—Used to package lip balm and deodorant.

Label Maker or Craft Labels—Always label your creations with product names and ingredients using either printable labels or handwritten craft labels. Used for all recipes as needed.

TIP: I consider my label maker to be the "MVP" of my equipment arsenal. I don't know what I would do without it! When you're making an item, you may think you'll easily remember what's in the bottle, but trust me, you never do! Label things as soon as you bottle them.

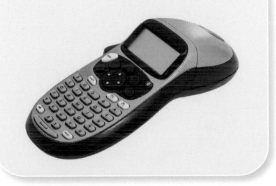

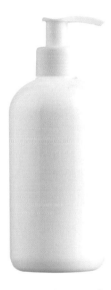

Pump or Squeeze Bottles—A glass, aluminum, or plastic bottle with a pump top or soft plastic bottles that allow for squeezing to expel the product. Used to package lotions, cream cleansers, and body and massage oils.

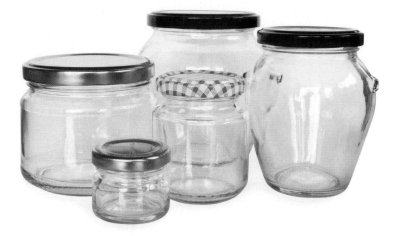

Recycled Jars (of all kinds)—Used to package
scrubs, lotions, creams, and cleansers.

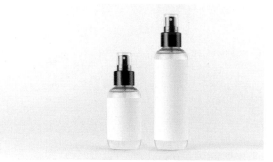

**Spray Bottles (1-ounce, 2-ounce, 4-ounce,
8-ounce, 16-ounce)**—Used to package toners,
face mists, cleansers, and cleaning products.

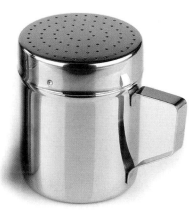

Shaker Tube or Can—These metal, paper, or
plastic tubes/canisters have perforated tops that
allow for the shaking out of powdered products.
Used to package dry shampoo and carpet cleaner.

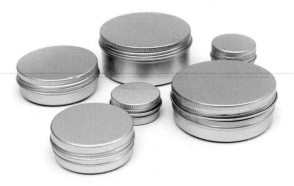

Tins (1-ounce, 2-ounce, 4-ounce)—Used to
package balms, butters, salves, and creams.

Wax Paper Bags and Decorative Papers—Used
to package soaps.

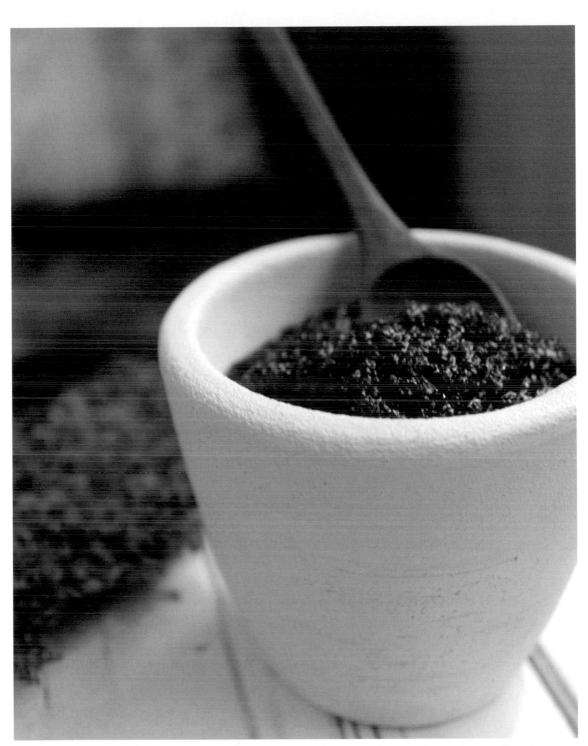

Customizing your own scrubs is one of the most enjoyable parts of making self-care products at home. Adjust the type and amount of exfoliants used in my Oceana Sands Scrub on page 114 to suit your preferences.

PART 5

Blends for Health and Healing

This section features recipes for two types of pure aromatherapy blends—mood-improving oil blends and blends with more specific, medicinal uses. The mood-improving blends all feature two variations so you can get the same benefits from the essential oils with the fragrances you most prefer. Blending for medicinal purposes is slightly different from blending for mood benefits, as the aroma is secondary to the healing benefits of the oils. Some may smell strong or medicinal, but that often means the oils are doing their work!

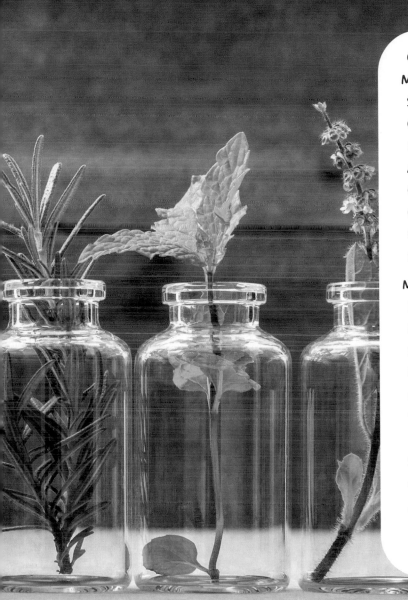

Culinary herbs also offer mood and medicinal healing
via their pure, extracted essential oils.

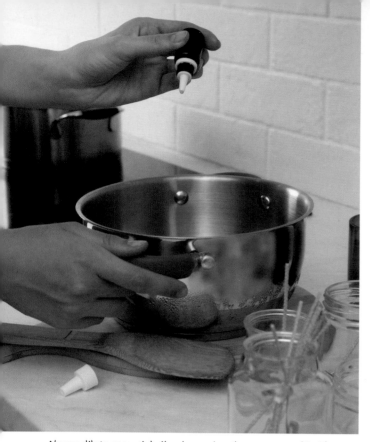

The underlying philosophy of aromatherapy and essential oil therapy is that plant essential oils have similar biochemical effects on humans to those they have within the plants. Essential oils can, of course, be mixed with other self-care ingredients to create cleansers, masks, candles, sprays, and other products that make use of these properties, but one of the easiest ways to begin introducing essential oils into your life is to develop and use oil blends diluted with a simple carrier oil or other liquid.

All recipes in this section are written for carrier oil–diluted topical application via a dropper, nozzle, or roller ball bottle. To use in a diffuser, omit the carrier oil and add the essential oils directly to your diffuser. To use as a mist, replace the carrier oil with perfumer's alcohol or your liquid of choice (hydrosol, witch hazel, etc.) and use a mister or spray bottle. (If you use hydrosol, refrigerate your product or add a preservative.) See 20 Quick Ways to Incorporate Essential Oils into Your Life on page 21 for more ideas.

Always dilute essential oils when using them on your skin. There are many dispersant options, including carrier oils, floral waters, balms, and creams.

SAFE DILUTION AND APPLICATION

Remember, essential oils are not safe to ingest or use directly on the skin. When applied topically, they should always be diluted in a carrier oil or other liquid. Proper dilution ranges between 2–10 percent, depending on your blend's purpose and the specific oils you're using. For example, in a 15ml bottle, which can hold approximately 300 drops total, your essential oils should be only about 6–15 drops of the total mixture. The rest would be a carrier oil or other liquid. **THE RECIPES IN THIS SECTION USE A 5 PERCENT DILUTION. IF YOU HAVE SENSITIVE SKIN, REDUCE ACCORDINGLY.**

Also, each of us is unique in our reactions to essential oils, so be sure to "patch test" a bit of diluted oil on a small area of skin to confirm you won't have a bad reaction before using it in your blends. If an oil doesn't work for you, simply substitute it with a similar oil that does work!

CUSTOMIZING YOUR OWN BLENDS

A harmonious blend typically has top, middle, and base notes. The top note is the first to hit the nose, and the first to dissipate. Top notes include citrus oils and some lighter herbs and woods, like eucalyptus and rosemary. The middle note is the heart of the blend, the oil you may want to use the most of. It's often a favorite, such as lavender, clary sage, or rose. The base note will linger the longest on the skin and can often overpower a blend—so it's used in the smallest quantity. Base notes are typically woods like vetiver, cinnamon bark, and cedar but may also be strong flowers like jasmine and ylang ylang. Some blends made solely for certain health or mood effects might not have all three notes, but having a top, middle, and base note is a standard in perfumery for creating complex and long-lasting blends.

See Getting Started—The Most *Essential* Essential Oils on page 14 and Recommended Essential Oils on page 17 for details on the benefits of some of the most popular oils, and remember that there are hundreds of other

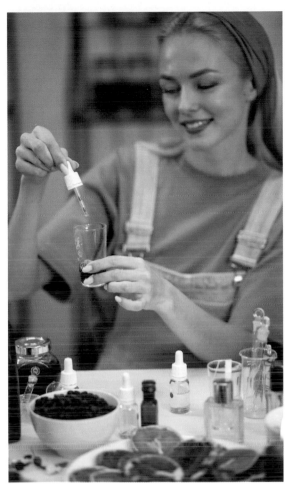

Blending is both art and science. After learning a few basic principles, play around with your oils to get a feel for what you like best.

essential oils available that offer other benefits. I encourage you to explore and experiment with them all—our reactions to essential oils are very personal and if you don't like something in one of the blends in this chapter, simply substitute an essential oil that provides the same benefits, but with a scent you love. And remember, just like any good sauce recipe, the essential oils will continue to marinate after you've mixed them— your aroma will pleasantly evolve over time!

TIP: Avoid wasting oils or creating a blend you don't love by checking the scent combinations first! Open and move the essential oil bottles under your nose and inhale deeply to see how you react to the blended aromas. You'll get a good sense of whether you've got a winning combination before ever mixing any of your precious oils.

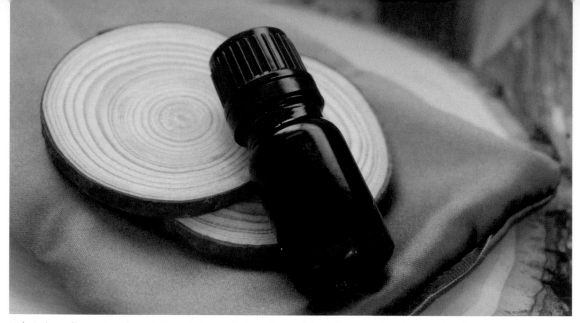

Help induce sleep naturally with the calming, sedative effects of these flower and grass essential oils.

SLEEP SUPPORT

Many people have trouble relaxing once it's time to go to bed. These two blend options are soothing and have sedative properties—helping you more easily achieve a peaceful night's sleep. Authentic sandalwood essential oil is quite expensive, so if you're making that variation and don't have any on hand, feel free to substitute it with another wood or resin oil, like vetiver, myrrh, or cedar.

EQUIPMENT

- ½-ounce (15ml) dark glass dropper bottle
- Pipettes
- Funnel
- Glass measuring cup

INGREDIENTS

Base:
- Carrier oil of choice

Essential Oils, Variation 1:
- 9 drops lavender
- 5 drops neroli
- 1 drop citronella

Essential Oils, Variation 2:
- 7 drops sandalwood
- 4 drops rose otto (or rose in jojoba)
- 4 drops lemon verbena

HOW TO MAKE

1. Remove the plastic dropper tops from your essential oil bottles. **Note:** If you choose to leave on the dropper nozzles, you can still shake the required number of drops into the blending bottle; it will just be a bit harder to control the accuracy.
2. Place your funnel over your bottle and add each essential oil one at a time with pipettes.
3. Still using the funnel, fill the remainder of the bottle with your chosen carrier oil, leaving a bit of room at the top so the cap does not cause any overflow. Cap and swirl gently to blend.

HOW TO USE

Drop or roll the blended oils onto your wrists or massage into the skin of your hands, feet, neck, chest, ears, or anywhere you like. Breathe in deeply to enjoy the benefits of each essential oil. See page 21 for additional use ideas.

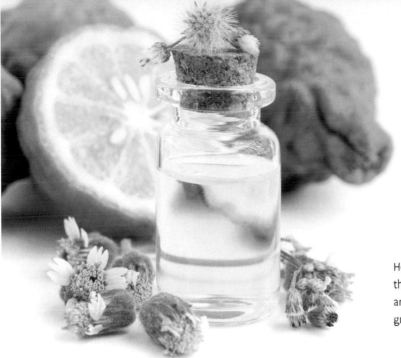

Heart-soothing oils help take the edge off the pain of grief and connect us to a feeling of grounded safety.

GRIEF RELIEF

The variation of this blend made with rose and white pine was my first introduction to the power of essential oils (see page 8). Florals mixed with a deep woodsy base help us feel grounded and comforted.

EQUIPMENT
- ½-ounce (15ml) dark glass dropper bottle
- Pipettes
- Funnel
- Glass measuring cup

INGREDIENTS
Base:
- Carrier oil of choice

Essential Oils, Variation 1:
- 9 drops rose otto (or use rose in jojoba for a more economical option)
- 6 drops white or Scotch pine

Essential Oils, Variation 2:
- 8 drops lavender
- 6 drops lime
- 1 drop vetiver

HOW TO MAKE
1. Remove the plastic dropper tops from your essential oil bottles. **Note:** If you choose to leave on the dropper nozzles, you can still shake the required number of drops into the blending bottle; it will just be a bit harder to control the accuracy.
2. Place your funnel over your bottle and add each essential oil one at a time with pipettes.
3. Still using the funnel, fill the remainder of the bottle with your chosen carrier oil, leaving a bit of room at the top so the cap does not cause any overflow. Cap and swirl gently to blend.

HOW TO USE
Drop or roll the blended oils onto your wrists or massage into the skin of your hands, feet, neck, chest, ears, or anywhere you like. Breathe in deeply to enjoy the benefits of each essential oil. See page 21 for additional use ideas.

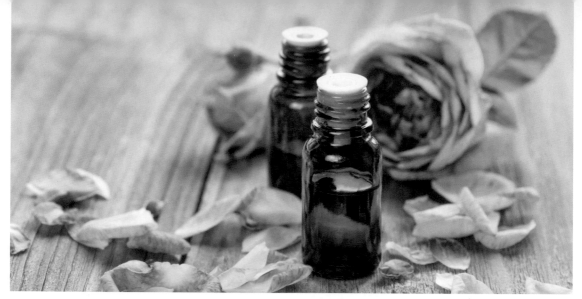

Rose essential oil can be expensive, but its mood-lifting qualities are worth every penny.

MOOD LIFT

You can take your blends in a few different directions if you're trying to create a blend that will boost your mood. Citrus is always a great choice if you want something joyful and energizing. You can also lean into bright, refreshing lemongrass and mint, softened with a floral note, for a completely different take on liquid joy!

EQUIPMENT

- ½-ounce (15ml) dark glass dropper bottle
- Pipettes
- Funnel
- Glass measuring cup

INGREDIENTS

Base:
- Carrier oil of choice

Essential Oils, Variation 1:
- 7 drops yuzu
- 6 drops lemon myrtle
- 2 drops ylang ylang

Essential Oils, Variation 2:
- 6 drops lemongrass
- 4 drops rose
- 3 drops peppermint

HOW TO MAKE

1. Remove the plastic dropper tops from your essential oil bottles. **Note:** If you choose to leave on the dropper nozzles, you can still shake the required number of drops into the blending bottle; it will just be a bit harder to control the accuracy.
2. Place your funnel over your bottle and add each essential oil one at a time with pipettes.
3. Still using the funnel, fill the remainder of the bottle with your chosen carrier oil, leaving a bit of room at the top so the cap does not cause any overflow. Cap and swirl gently to blend.

HOW TO USE

Drop or roll the blended oils onto your wrists or massage into the skin of your hands, feet, neck, chest, ears, or anywhere you like. Breathe in deeply to enjoy the benefits of each essential oil. See page 21 for additional use ideas.

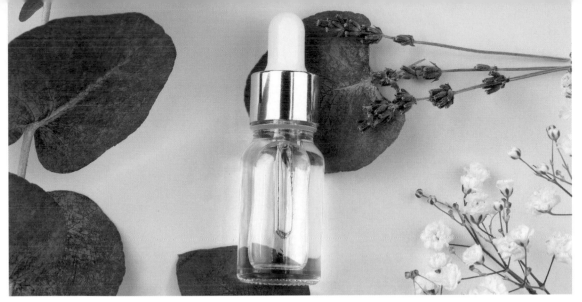

Sweet citrus, deep wood scents, and floral notes combine to soothe an anxious mind.

ANTIANXIETY

Both of these variations have sweet citrus top notes that combine with the other scents to calm us in our tensest of moments. Authentic sandalwood essential oil is quite expensive; feel free to substitute it with another wood or resin oil, like vetiver, balsam copaiba or black spruce.

EQUIPMENT
- ½-ounce (15ml) dark glass dropper bottle
- Pipettes
- Funnel
- Glass measuring cup

INGREDIENTS
Base:
- Carrier oil of choice

Essential Oils, Variation 1:
- 6 drops sweet orange
- 6 drops rose otto
- 2 drops clary sage
- 1 drop cedarwood

Essential Oils, Variation 2:
- 6 drops pink grapefruit
- 5 drops sandalwood
- 4 drops lavender

HOW TO MAKE
1. Remove the plastic dropper tops from your essential oil bottles. **Note:** If you choose to leave on the dropper nozzles, you can still shake the required number of drops into the blending bottle; it will just be a bit harder to control the accuracy.
2. Place your funnel over your bottle and add each essential oil one at a time with pipettes.
3. Still using the funnel, fill the remainder of the bottle with your chosen carrier oil, leaving a bit of room at the top so the cap does not cause any overflow. Cap and swirl gently to blend.

HOW TO USE
Drop or roll the blended oils onto your wrists or massage into the skin of your hands, feet, neck, chest, ears, or anywhere you like. Breathe in deeply to enjoy the benefits of each essential oil. See page 21 for additional use ideas.

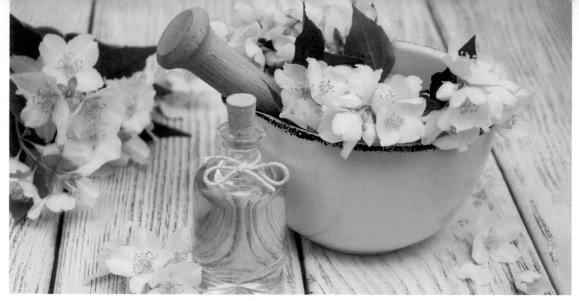

Both of these variations combine light floral notes with woody base notes like black spruce and vetiver.

GROUNDING

Grounding softens challenging emotions and thoughts, bringing us back to our best selves. Smell is one of the most powerful tools for grounding, and these scent combinations will help you effectively refocus on the present.

EQUIPMENT

- ½-ounce (15ml) dark glass dropper bottle
- Pipettes
- Funnel
- Glass measuring cup

INGREDIENTS

Base:
- Carrier oil of choice

Essential Oils, Variation 1:
- 6 drops black spruce
- 3 drops rose otto
- 2 drops jasmine
- 2 drops ylang ylang

Essential Oils, Variation 2:
- 9 drops sweet orange
- 4 drops lavender
- 1 drop vetiver

HOW TO MAKE

1. Remove the plastic dropper tops from your essential oil bottles. **Note:** If you choose to leave on the dropper nozzles, you can still shake the required number of drops into the blending bottle; it will just be a bit harder to control the accuracy.
2. Place your funnel over your bottle and add each essential oil one at a time with pipettes.
3. Still using the funnel, fill the remainder of the bottle with your chosen carrier oil, leaving a bit of room at the top so the cap does not cause any overflow. Cap and swirl gently to blend.

HOW TO USE

Drop or roll the blended oils onto your wrists or massage into the skin of your hands, feet, neck, chest, ears, or anywhere you like. Breathe in deeply to enjoy the benefits of each essential oil. See page 21 for additional use ideas.

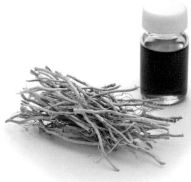

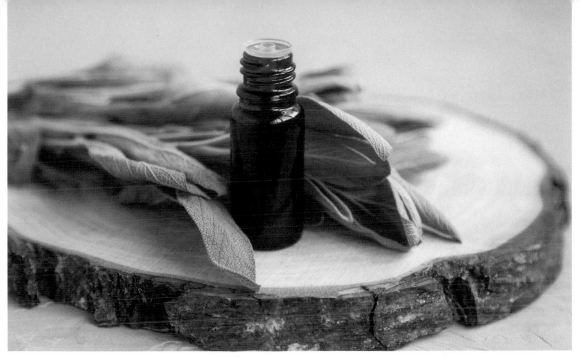

The first variation blends warm, savory sage with eucalyptus and lemon verbena to soothe and lift the spirits.

OPTIMISM

Fresh citrus and bright herbal scents combine perfectly to inspire an uplifting sense of optimism.

EQUIPMENT

- ½ ounce (15ml) dark glass dropper bottle
- Pipettes
- Funnel
- Glass measuring cup

INGREDIENTS

Base:
- Carrier oil of choice

Essential Oils, Variation 1:
- 8 drops lemon verbena
- 5 drops eucalyptus
- 2 drops sage

Essential Oils, Variation 2:
- 8 drops bergamot
- 4 drops juniper berry
- 3 drops tangerine

HOW TO MAKE

1. Remove the plastic dropper tops from your essential oil bottles. **Note:** If you choose to leave on the dropper nozzles, you can still shake the required number of drops into the blending bottle; it will just be a bit harder to control the accuracy.
2. Place your funnel over your bottle and add each essential oil one at a time with pipettes.
3. Still using the funnel, fill the remainder of the bottle with your chosen carrier oil, leaving a bit of room at the top so the cap does not cause any overflow. Cap and swirl gently to blend.

HOW TO USE

Drop or roll the blended oils onto your wrists or massage into the skin of your hands, feet, neck, chest, ears, or anywhere you like. Breathe in deeply to enjoy the benefits of each essential oil. See page 21 for additional use ideas.

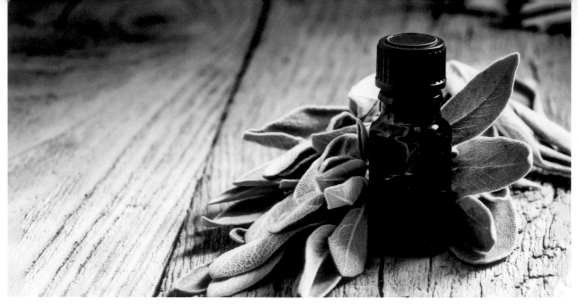

Clary sage essential oil adds an earthy quality to the complex second variation of this blend.

CONTENTMENT

A sense of gratitude and satisfaction is often the first step in any healing journey. These scents help promote that welcome feeling of contented happiness.

EQUIPMENT

- ½-ounce (15ml) dark glass dropper bottle
- Pipettes
- Funnel
- Glass measuring cup

INGREDIENTS

Base:
- Carrier oil of choice

Essential Oils, Variation 1:
- 10 drops geranium rose
- 3 drops sweet marjoram
- 2 drops jasmine

Essential Oils, Variation 2:
- 5 drops lavender
- 4 drops clary sage
- 4 drops bergamot
- 2 drops frankincense

HOW TO MAKE

1. Remove the plastic dropper tops from your essential oil bottles. **Note:** If you choose to leave on the dropper nozzles, you can still shake the required number of drops into the blending bottle; it will just be a bit harder to control the accuracy.
2. Place your funnel over your bottle and add each essential oil one at a time with pipettes.
3. Still using the funnel, fill the remainder of the bottle with your chosen carrier oil, leaving a bit of room at the top so the cap does not cause any overflow. Cap and swirl gently to blend.

HOW TO USE

Drop or roll the blended oils onto your wrists or massage into the skin of your hands, feet, neck, chest, ears, or anywhere you like. Breathe in deeply to enjoy the benefits of each essential oil. See page 21 for additional use ideas.

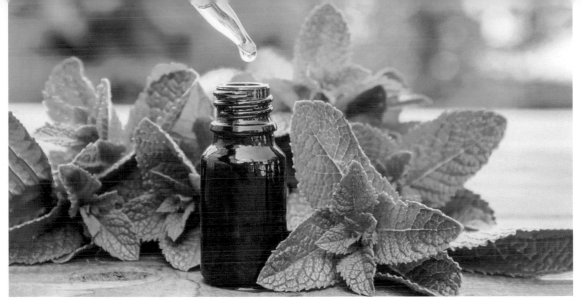

Peppermint is an accessible oil that brings energy and a more focused mind.

ENERGY

Citrus oils and mentholic peppermint naturally invigorate the senses. If you're having trouble waking up or just need an afternoon boost, these blend options are for you.

EQUIPMENT
- ½-ounce (15ml) dark glass dropper bottle
- Pipettes
- Funnel
- Glass measuring cup

INGREDIENTS
Base:
- Carrier oil of choice

Essential Oils, Variation 1:
- 8 drops peppermint
- 4 drops lemon
- 3 drops eucalyptus

Essential Oils, Variation 2:
- 9 drops sweet orange
- 5 drops bergamot
- 1 drop rosemary

HOW TO MAKE
1. Remove the plastic dropper tops from your essential oil bottles. **Note:** If you choose to leave on the dropper nozzles, you can still shake the required number of drops into the blending bottle; it will just be a bit harder to control the accuracy.
2. Place your funnel over your bottle and add each essential oil one at a time with pipettes.
3. Still using the funnel, fill the remainder of the bottle with your chosen carrier oil, leaving a bit of room at the top so the cap does not cause any overflow. Cap and swirl gently to blend.

HOW TO USE
Drop or roll the blended oils onto your wrists or massage into the skin of your hands, feet, neck, chest, ears, or anywhere you like. Breathe in deeply to enjoy the benefits of each essential oil. See page 21 for additional use ideas.

BE WELL

This blend is strongly antibacterial and antiviral, and acts as a decongestant, antiseptic, and disinfectant. Use it when you're under the weather or feel something coming on.

EQUIPMENT
- ½-ounce (15ml) dark glass dropper bottle
- Pipettes
- Funnel
- Glass measuring cup

INGREDIENTS
Base:
- Carrier oil of choice

Essential Oils:
- 6 drops lemon
- 4 drops eucalyptus
- 3 drops juniper berry
- 2 drops tea tree

HOW TO MAKE
1. Remove the plastic dropper tops from your essential oil bottles. **Note:** If you choose to leave on the dropper nozzles, you can still shake the required number of drops into the blending bottle; it will just be a bit harder to control the accuracy.
2. Place your funnel over your bottle and add each essential oil one at a time with pipettes.
3. Still using the funnel, fill the remainder of the bottle with your chosen carrier oil, leaving a bit of room at the top so the cap does not cause any overflow. Cap and swirl gently to blend.

HOW TO USE
I like to use this type of blend in the shower, to breathe in deeply with the steam. See page 21 for additional use ideas.

HEADACHE REMEDY

There are few everyday ailments quite as distressing as a headache that just won't go away. This blend has pain-relieving essential oils and scents that help to clear the sinuses and release some of the tensions that cause many of the most common types of headaches.

EQUIPMENT
- ½-ounce (15ml) dark glass dropper bottle
- Pipettes
- Funnel
- Glass measuring cup

INGREDIENTS
Base:
- Carrier oil of choice

Essential Oils:
- 6 drops lavender
- 4 drops peppermint
- 4 drops eucalyptus
- 1 drop rosemary

HOW TO MAKE
1. Remove the plastic dropper tops from your essential oil bottles. **Note:** If you choose to leave on the dropper nozzles, you can still shake the required number of drops into the blending bottle; it will just be a bit harder to control the accuracy.
2. Place your funnel over your bottle and add each essential oil one at a time with pipettes.
3. Still using the funnel, fill the remainder of the bottle with your chosen carrier oil, leaving a bit of room at the top so the cap does not cause any overflow. Cap and swirl gently to blend.

HOW TO USE
Use this remedy on your temples, under your nose, or on a soothing warm washcloth before laying down to relax and breathe. You can also massage it directly into your temples, on the back of your neck, or anywhere you feel pain.

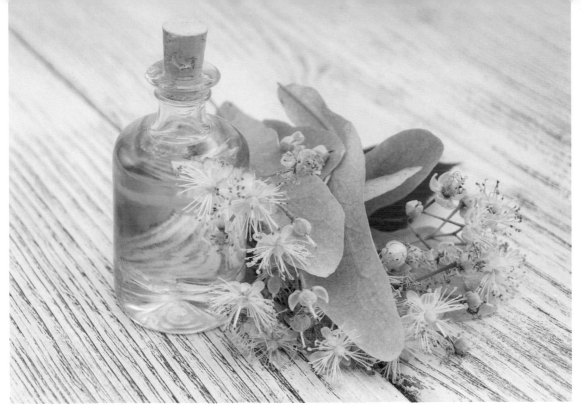

Lemon myrtle combines many of the benefits of citrus and floral scents in one essential oil.

PAIN BE GONE

Essential oils are part of the immune system of a plant and can have similar benefits for us. Try the below recipe to ease pain in any area.

EQUIPMENT
- ½-ounce (15ml) dark glass dropper bottle
- Pipettes
- Funnel
- Glass measuring cup

INGREDIENTS
Base:
- Carrier oil of choice

Essential Oils:
- 6 drops lavender
- 5 drops lemon myrtle
- 2 drops chamomile
- 2 drops rosemary

HOW TO MAKE
1. Remove the plastic dropper tops from your essential oil bottles. **Note:** If you choose to leave on the dropper nozzles, you can still shake the required number of drops into the blending bottle; it will just be a bit harder to control the accuracy.
2. Place your funnel over your bottle and add each essential oil one at a time with pipettes.
3. Still using the funnel, fill the remainder of the bottle with your chosen carrier oil, leaving a bit of room at the top so the cap does not cause any overflow. Cap and swirl gently to blend.

HOW TO USE
Massage directly onto sore muscles, bruises, bug bites or wherever needed.

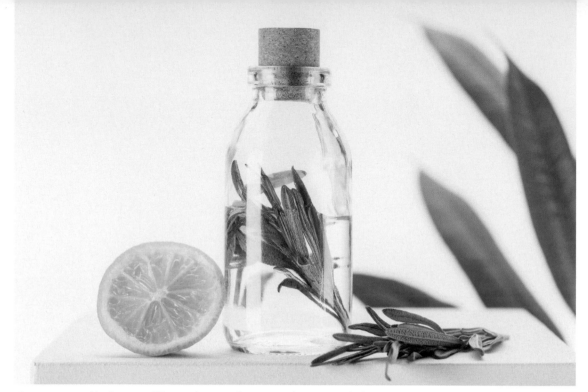

Citrus scents and herbs are well known bug repellents. Try other herbal oils, like rosemary, for a variation.

BUG SHOO

Be sure to pack this natural bug repellant when you're out camping, picnicking, or eating al fresco. This blend also works well as a mist.

EQUIPMENT

- ½-ounce (15ml) dark glass dropper bottle
- Pipettes
- Funnel
- Glass measuring cup

INGREDIENTS

Base:
- Carrier oil of choice

Essential Oils:
- 8 drops citronella
- 6 drops lemon
- 1 drop thyme

HOW TO MAKE

1. Remove the plastic dropper tops from your essential oil bottles. **Note:** If you choose to leave on the dropper nozzles, you can still shake the required number of drops into the blending bottle; it will just be a bit harder to control the accuracy.
2. Place your funnel over your bottle and add each essential oil one at a time with pipettes.
3. Still using the funnel, fill the remainder of the bottle with your chosen carrier oil, leaving a bit of room at the top so the cap does not cause any overflow. Cap and swirl gently to blend.

HOW TO USE

Drop the blend onto picnic tables, into candles, or massage it into your skin. If you make this blend as a mist, spray it onto exposed skin.

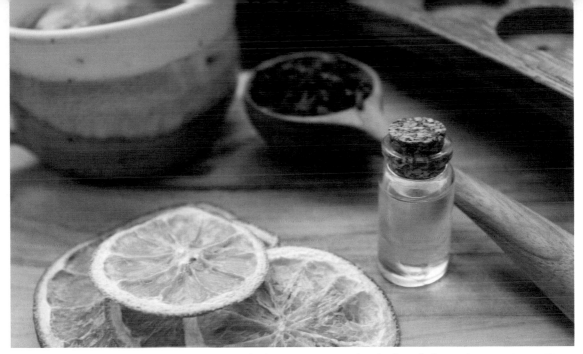

I keep this little bottle in my medicine chest and dab a bit on my wrists and neck when I feel something coming on. You can also skip the carrier oil and drop the essential oils directly into your diffuser to breathe in the oils' healing benefits.

FLU BUSTER

Clove bud and sweet orange essential oils both have powerful antiviral properties to help protect you during the cold and flu season. They will work in your favor if a virus is in your midst!

EQUIPMENT

- ½-ounce (15ml) dark glass dropper bottle
- Pipettes
- Funnel
- Glass measuring cup

INGREDIENTS

Base:
- Carrier oil of choice

Essential Oils:
- 8 drops sweet orange
- 6 drops bergamot
- 1 drop clove bud

HOW TO MAKE

1. Remove the plastic dropper tops from your essential oil bottles. **Note:** If you choose to leave on the dropper nozzles, you can still shake the required number of drops into the blending bottle; it will just be a bit harder to control the accuracy.
2. Place your funnel over your bottle and add each essential oil one at a time with pipettes.
3. Still using the funnel, fill the remainder of the bottle with your chosen carrier oil, leaving a bit of room at the top so the cap does not cause any overflow. Cap and swirl gently to blend.

HOW TO USE

Dab onto your wrists and inhale deeply; or, if you're already sick, drop into a steaming bowl of water, cover your head with a towel, and breathe in for a couple of minutes.

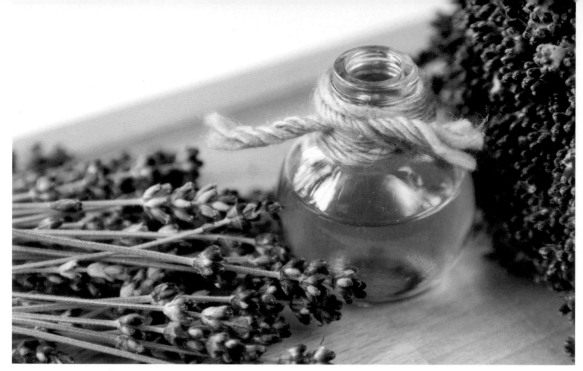

Give yourself natural protection when traveling or in large crowds.

IMMUNITY BOOST

On days where you feel the need for a bit more protection from assaults on your immune system, use the naturally boosting chemicals found in these essential oils. A must-use item for traveling!

EQUIPMENT
- ½-ounce (15ml) dark glass dropper bottle
- Pipettes
- Funnel
- Glass measuring cup

INGREDIENTS
Base:
- Carrier oil of choice

Essential Oils:
- 11 drops lavender
- 3 drops eucalyptus
- 1 drop tea tree

HOW TO MAKE
1. Remove the plastic dropper tops from your essential oil bottles. **Note:** If you choose to leave on the dropper nozzles, you can still shake the required number of drops into the blending bottle; it will just be a bit harder to control the accuracy.
2. Place your funnel over your bottle and add each essential oil one at a time with pipettes.
3. Still using the funnel, fill the remainder of the bottle with your chosen carrier oil, leaving a bit of room at the top so the cap does not cause any overflow. Cap and swirl gently to blend.

HOW TO USE
Drop or roll the blended oils onto your wrists or massage into the skin of your hands, feet, neck, chest, ears, or anywhere you like. Breathe in deeply to enjoy the benefits of each essential oil. See page 21 for additional use ideas.

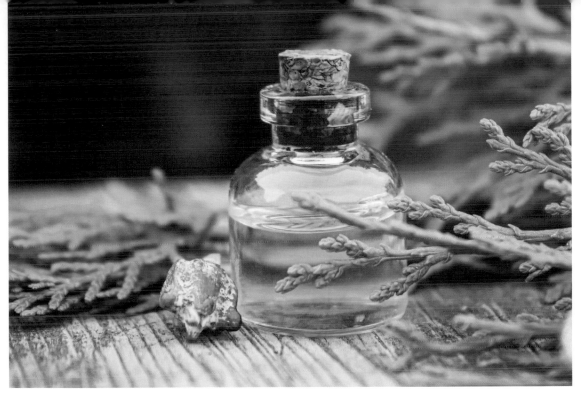

Cypress essential oil can clear your mind as well as your sinuses. It has a beautiful, foresty scent.

BREATHE EASY SINUS CLEAR

Trees are often called the earth's "lungs," absorbing pollutants and keeping our air clean. Cypress essential oil works similarly here as a natural decongestant on your own personal "ecosystem."

EQUIPMENT

- ½ ounce (15ml) dark glass dropper bottle
- Pipettes
- Funnel
- Glass measuring cup

INGREDIENTS

Base:
- Carrier oil of choice

Essential Oils:
- 8 drops cypress
- 5 drops eucalyptus
- 2 drops tea tree

HOW TO MAKE

1. Remove the plastic dropper tops from your essential oil bottles. **Note:** If you choose to leave on the dropper nozzles, you can still shake the required number of drops into the blending bottle; it will just be a bit harder to control the accuracy.
2. Place your funnel over your bottle and add each essential oil one at a time with pipettes.
3. Still using the funnel, fill the remainder of the bottle with your chosen carrier oil, leaving a bit of room at the top so the cap does not cause any overflow. Cap and swirl gently to blend.

HOW TO USE

Drop or roll the blended oils onto your wrists or massage into the skin of your hands, feet, neck, chest, ears, or anywhere you like. Breathe in deeply to enjoy the benefits of each essential oil. See page 21 for additional use ideas.

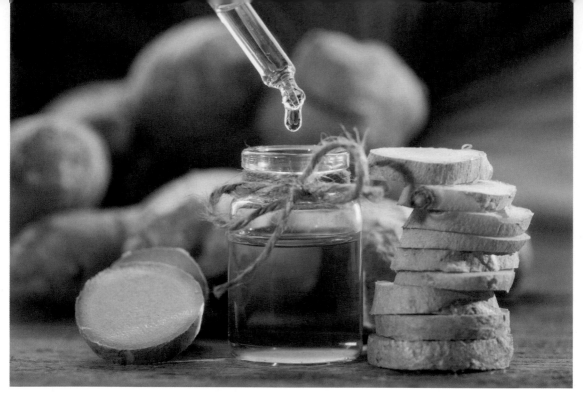

Ginger essential oil is the magic ingredient in this soothing blend.

STOMACH SOOTHE

Massage this blend into your abdomen to help resolve indigestion and stomach upset. You may also dab it under your nose and lay down to breathe the fragrance or drop only the undiluted essential oils into your diffuser and breathe in deeply.

EQUIPMENT

- ½-ounce (15ml) dark glass dropper bottle
- Pipettes
- Funnel
- Glass measuring cup

INGREDIENTS

Base:
- Carrier oil of choice

Essential Oils:
- 8 drops orange
- 3 drops lime
- 2 drops ginger

HOW TO MAKE

1. Remove the plastic dropper tops from your essential oil bottles.
   Note: If you choose to leave on the dropper nozzles, you can still shake the required number of drops into the blending bottle; it will just be a bit harder to control the accuracy.
2. Place your funnel over your bottle and add each essential oil one at a time with pipettes.
3. Still using the funnel, fill the remainder of the bottle with your chosen carrier oil, leaving a bit of room at the top so the cap does not cause any overflow. Cap and swirl gently to blend.

HOW TO USE

Drop or roll the blended oils onto your stomach or under your nose. Breathe in deeply to enjoy the benefits of each essential oil. See page 21 for additional use ideas.

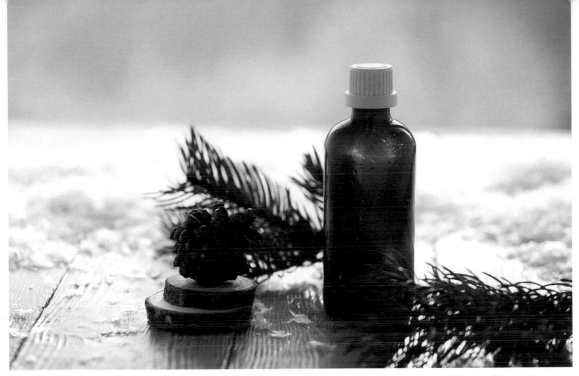

The majestic forest-like scent of pine and the fresh peppermint work together to open up your airways, allowing you to breathe more easily.

CHEST DECOMPRESS

This blend works wonderfully when dropped onto a steaming hot towel and placed over the chest before lying down. You can also drop the oils directly into a pot of steaming water, cover your head with a towel, and breathe in deeply for 2 to 3 minutes.

EQUIPMENT

- ½-ounce (15ml) dark glass dropper bottle
- Pipettes
- Funnel
- Glass measuring cup

INGREDIENTS

Base:
- Carrier oil of choice

Essential Oils:
- 7 drops peppermint
- 6 drops pine
- 2 drops marjoram

HOW TO MAKE

1. Remove the plastic dropper tops from your essential oil bottles.
   Note: If you choose to leave on the dropper nozzles, you can still shake the required number of drops into the blending bottle; it will just be a bit harder to control the accuracy.
2. Place your funnel over your bottle and add each essential oil one at a time with pipettes.
3. Still using the funnel, fill the remainder of the bottle with your chosen carrier oil, leaving a bit of room at the top so the cap does not cause any overflow. Cap and swirl gently to blend.

HOW TO USE

Combine the blended oils with steam, using a hot towel or a pot of water and breathe in deeply to enjoy the benefits of each essential oil. See page 21 for additional use ideas.

ARTHRITIS SUPPORT

These oils are analgesic and anti-inflammatory, working well to soothe sore, arthritic joints. Use daily on affected areas.

EQUIPMENT
- ½-ounce (15ml) dark glass dropper bottle
- Pipettes
- Funnel
- Glass measuring cup

INGREDIENTS
Base:
- Carrier oil of choice

Essential Oils:
- 8 drops frankincense
- 6 drops Roman chamomile
- 1 drop yarrow

HOW TO MAKE
1. Remove the plastic dropper tops from your essential oil bottles. **Note:** If you choose to leave on the dropper nozzles, you can still shake the required number of drops into the blending bottle; it will just be a bit harder to control the accuracy.
2. Place your funnel over your bottle and add each essential oil one at a time with pipettes.
3. Still using the funnel, fill the remainder of the bottle with your chosen carrier oil, leaving a bit of room at the top so the cap does not cause any overflow. Cap and swirl gently to blend.

HOW TO USE
Massage the blended oils into the skin of the affected area to enjoy the benefits of each essential oil. See page 21 for additional use ideas.

WOUND HEALING

Research shows that essential oils have chemical compounds that expedite healing when applied to the skin. For minor cuts and burns, integrate this blend into your self-care practice. I always have a bottle in my medicine chest.

EQUIPMENT
- ½-ounce (15ml) dark glass dropper bottle
- Pipettes
- Funnel
- Glass measuring cup

INGREDIENTS
Base:
- Carrier oil of choice

Essential Oils:
- 9 drops lavender
- 4 drops balsam copaiba
- 1 drop helichrysum

HOW TO MAKE
1. Remove the plastic dropper tops from your essential oil bottles. **Note:** If you choose to leave on the dropper nozzles, you can still shake the required number of drops into the blending bottle; it will just be a bit harder to control the accuracy.
2. Place your funnel over your bottle and add each essential oil one at a time with pipettes.
3. Still using the funnel, fill the remainder of the bottle with your chosen carrier oil, leaving a bit of room at the top so the cap does not cause any overflow. Cap and swirl gently to blend.

HOW TO USE
Apply these blended oils onto minor cuts and burns as needed to enjoy the benefits of each essential oil. See page 21 for additional use ideas.

HORMONE BALANCER

When you feel out of sorts and know the culprit is hormones, try this blend to wake up with an improved mood.

EQUIPMENT
- ½-ounce (15ml) dark glass dropper bottle
- Pipettes
- Funnel
- Glass measuring cup

INGREDIENTS
Base:
- Carrier oil of choice

Essential Oils:
- 5 drops clary sage
- 4 drops rose geranium
- 3 drops orange

HOW TO MAKE
1. Remove the plastic dropper tops from your essential oil bottles. **Note:** If you choose to leave on the dropper nozzles, you can still shake the required number of drops into the blending bottle; it will just be a bit harder to control the accuracy.
2. Place your funnel over your bottle and add each essential oil one at a time with pipettes.
3. Still using the funnel, fill the remainder of the bottle with your chosen carrier oil, leaving a bit of room at the top so the cap does not cause any overflow. Cap and swirl gently to blend.

HOW TO USE
Massage the blended oils onto your chest or place the pure essential oils into a diffuser on your nightstand at bedtime to enjoy the benefits of each essential oil. See page 21 for additional use ideas.

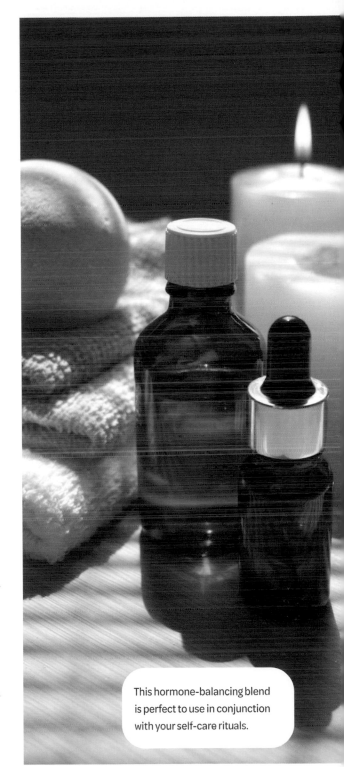

This hormone-balancing blend is perfect to use in conjunction with your self-care rituals.

PART 6

Recipes for Face, Body, and Home

Easily incorporate essential oils into your daily life with natural, pampering products for self-care. Without harmful chemicals, these recipes bring the power of plants to your mind, body, and home.

Bath bombs are a fun project to make at home, especially with children and friends. Start with the basic recipes on pages 162–167 and then experiment with your own scents, colors, and additives.

I chose the essential oils for each recipe based on their chemical profiles and benefits as well as their aromas, but feel free to substitute them with your favorites! I recommend checking the Essential Oil Chemical Families table on page 12 to ensure your final product provides the intended health benefits. You can also modify these recipes to substitute different types of carrier oils or clays, omit certain ingredients, etc.—most recipes will adapt easily. If you do modify a recipe, be sure to substitute a "like for like" ingredient—replace one type of clay with another type of clay, for example. Doing too much ingredient swapping can affect your results, so you'll want to mix and match carefully.

For lotions, substituting regular wax (beeswax or candelilla wax) for e-wax (emulsifying wax) will **not** work and you'll probably just end up with an impossible-to-clean mess in your blender. Without the proper ratios of ingredients, the cream may not emulsify. I recommend following emulsion (lotion) recipes exactly at first. Once you get a better feel for the process, you can begin to experiment with your own ratios and ingredient mixes.

Now, gather your ingredients and equipment and let's get started! I'm sending you all my best wishes for a beautiful bounty of hand-crafted treasures—and a lifetime of creative pleasure making your own beneficial products.

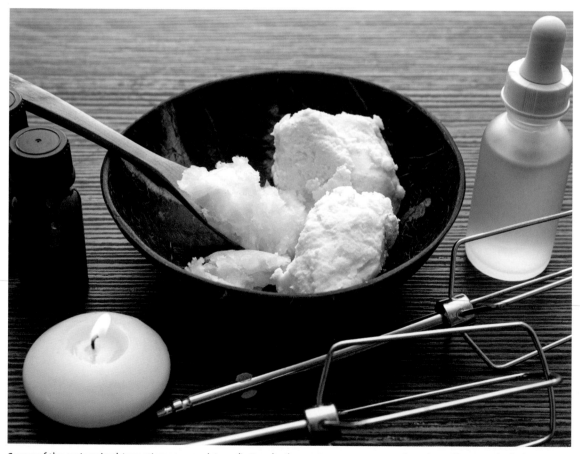

Some of the recipes in this section are emulsions (lotions)—there are separate water phase ingredients and oil phase ingredients. See page 67 for more information.

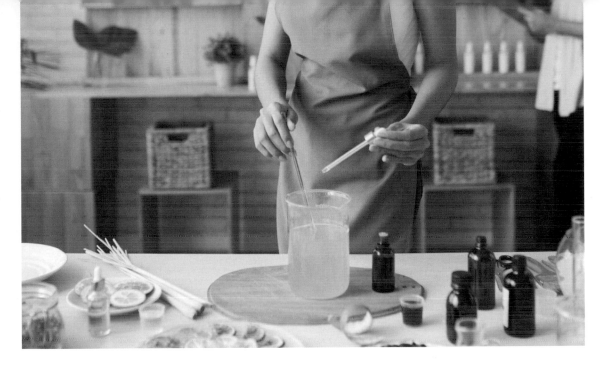

THE EMULSION PROCESS

Many of the cream-based products, such as the Rose Tea Cream Cleanser on page 76 and the Grapefruit Light Lotion on page 92, are emulsions, so they need to be specially mixed in phases. You'll begin by preparing the water phase and bringing it to the proper temperature, then you'll prepare the oil phase separately and bring it to the proper temperature. The final part of the process is blending the two phases together, lowering the temperature, and adding your essential oils and preservative.

Sticking to the proper temperatures and recipe step order will ensure success when making emulsion recipes, but you can also use the tips to the right to truly perfect your process.

Emulsion Tips

- For best results when making emulsions, weigh out your ingredients on a scale for accuracy.
- If you prefer, you can heat the water in a sanitized pot over low heat.

- For the water phase mixture, if you don't have a thermometer, simply test the temperature with a clean finger—it should feel very warm, almost hot.
- For the oil phase mixture, if you don't have a thermometer, swirl it around a bit and then touch the side of the glass bowl (or the stir stick) to test the temperature. You don't want to dip your finger in hot oil.
- If either the water phase mixture or oil phase mixture is much hotter than the other, place the hotter mixture in the freezer for a couple minutes. Check it often and remove once the temperatures are similar and within the 160°F–170°F (71°–77°C) range.
- Don't overblend. It can add a lot of air bubbles to the lotion, causing you to have very little product to fill your containers (for example, filling a 4-ounce bottle with only 1 ounce of actual product).

Rather than spending a huge amount of money on commercial products that contain chemicals, we can simply make beautiful, purely natural, plant-based products at home that leave our skin soft, radiant, and clear.

FACE CARE RECIPES

We interact with others and present ourselves to the world using our faces, so it's no wonder humans have been experimenting with lotions, potions, and makeups to beautify face skin since time immemorial. Beautiful skin largely comes from within, from healthy eating and getting plenty of water and exercise, but the recipes included here for cleansers, scrubs, toners, mists, masks, and moisturizers will naturally enhance the health of your face with organic botanical ingredients that make your skin glow—without chemical byproducts or wasteful packaging!

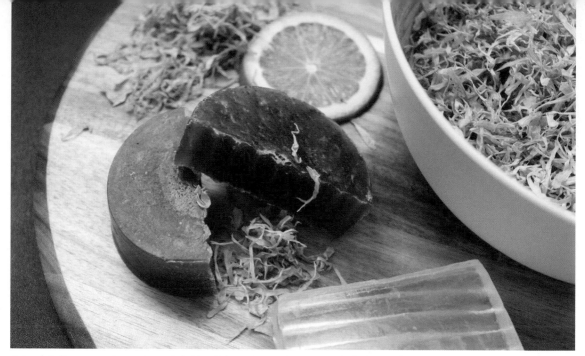

Calendula flower petals soothe and clarify, while sweet orange essential oil offers a cleansing vibrancy.

CALENDULA FACE BAR

FOR ALL SKIN TYPES ○ MAKES TWO 4-OUNCE (113G) BARS

Healing, soothing, and clarifying, this organic glycerin bar cleans and nourishes all skin types with antioxidant-rich calendula flower petals, which offer nutrients and gentle exfoliation. Additions include skin-regulating argan oil, kaolin clay for gentle extraction, vitamin C–rich orange peel powder, and optional vitamin E oil. The monoterpene-rich and vibrant orange essential oil offers antibacterial and detoxifying properties and lends a sweet, fresh scent. This lovely bar will keep your skin naturally clean and clear without chemicals or colorants.

EQUIPMENT

- Glass measuring cup
- Kitchen scale
- Two 4-ounce (113g) soap molds (round, oval, rectangular, or shape of choosing)
- Wooden stir stick or stirring spoon
- Wax paper, optional

INGREDIENTS

Base:
- 8 ounces (226g) clear glycerin soap blocks

Additives:
- 3 tablespoons (45ml) calendula flower petals
- ⅛ teaspoon (0.5ml) orange peel powder or dried orange zest
- ⅛ teaspoon (0.5ml) Moroccan red clay

- 6 drops argan oil
- 6 drops vitamin E oil, optional

Essential Oils:
- 2 teaspoons (10ml) sweet orange

Optional:
- ½ teaspoon (2.5ml) pink grapefruit
- ½ teaspoon (2.5ml) tangerine
- 3 drops ylang ylang

HOW TO MAKE

1. Weigh the glycerin soap blocks and cut them into ½" (1.3cm) cubes.
2. Place cut soap into the glass measuring cup and microwave, 1 minute at a time, stirring in between, until it is almost entirely melted.
3. Stir glycerin gently until it's fully melted.
4. Stir in the additives and essential oils, blending thoroughly.
5. Pour into the soap molds and let sit to cool. Wait at least 2 hours, then place in the freezer for 20 minutes.
6. Pop the bars out of the molds onto wax paper or a cutting board.

HOW TO USE

Gently massage into your skin and rinse with warm water, then pat dry. Follow with toner and hydration of choice.

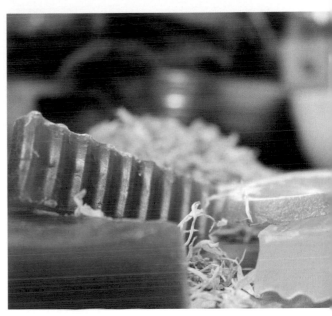

Infusing your glycerin soap with calendula petals is a quick and easy way to create a customized facial soap that naturally cleans and clarifies while providing gentle exfoliation and antioxidants.

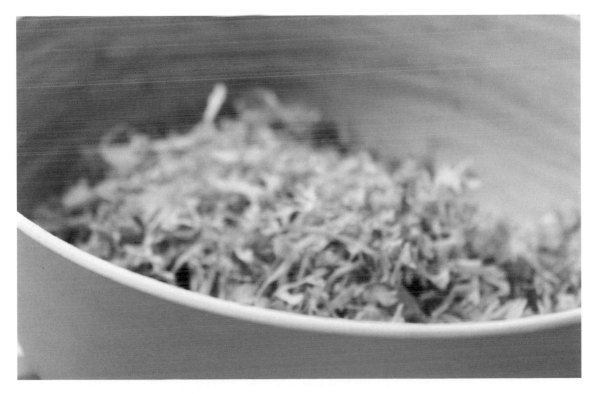

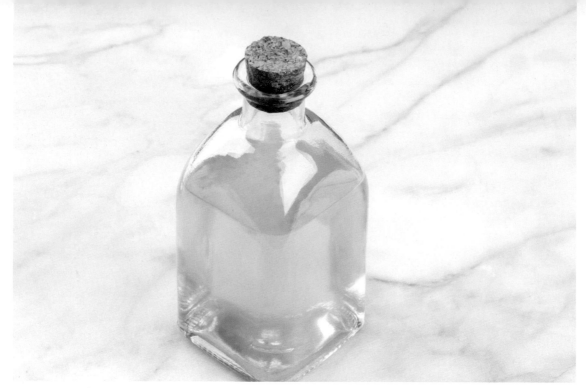

Using pure rose hydrosol instead of stronger rose essential oil creates a gentle cleanser perfect for any skin type.

ROSEWATER FACE WASH
FOR ALL SKIN TYPES ∘ MAKES 8 OUNCES (250ML)

This gentle cleansing splash features the healing botanicals of pure rose hydrosol, a bit of natural castile soap for cleansing, and glycerin for its moisturizing qualities, which hold the ingredients on your skin until they are absorbed. Light, lovely, and gentle for even the most sensitive skin.

EQUIPMENT
- Glass measuring cup
- 8-ounce (250ml) glass bottle with top
- Wooden stir stick or stirring spoon

INGREDIENTS
Base:
- 8 ounces (240ml) rose hydrosol
- 1½ teaspoon (7ml) glycerin
- 1½ teaspoon (7ml) castile soap

HOW TO MAKE
1. Pour all ingredients into glass measuring cup and stir.
2. Pour into glass bottle, replace top, and shake to mix.

HOW TO USE
Gently shake to reincorporate the ingredients, then place 1 to 2 teaspoons (5 to 10ml) into the palm of your hand. Splash onto your face, and massage the cleanser in. Rinse with warm water and pat dry. Follow with toner and hydration of choice.

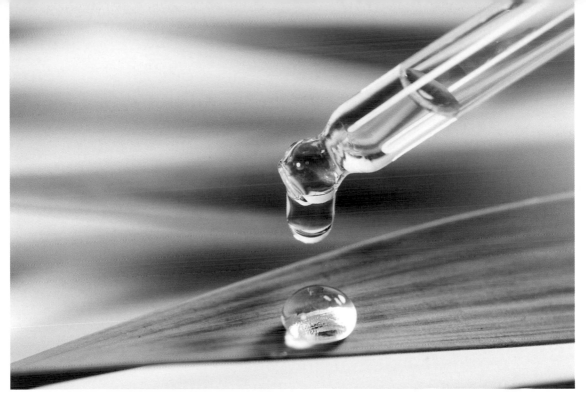

Tea tree essential oil has well-known antibacterial properties that help heal blemished skin.

TEA TREE CLARIFYING FACE WASH

FOR OILY SKIN ○ MAKES 8 OUNCES (250ML)

For oily or blemished skin, the antibacterial qualities of this refreshing tea tree cleanser help heal and clarify.

EQUIPMENT

- Glass measuring cup
- 8-ounce (250ml) glass bottle with top
- Wooden stir stick or stirring spoon

INGREDIENTS

Base:
- 8 ounces (250ml) tea tree hydrosol
- 1½ teaspoons (7ml) glycerin
- 1½ teaspoons (7ml) castile soap

Essential Oil
- 12 drops tea tree, optional

HOW TO MAKE

1. Pour all ingredients into glass measuring cup and stir.
2. Pour into glass bottle through funnel and swirl to mix. Cap.

HOW TO USE

Gently shake to reincorporate, and then place 1 to 2 teaspoons (5 to 10ml) into the palm of your hand. Splash onto your face and massage in. Rinse with warm water and pat dry. Follow with toner and hydration of choice.

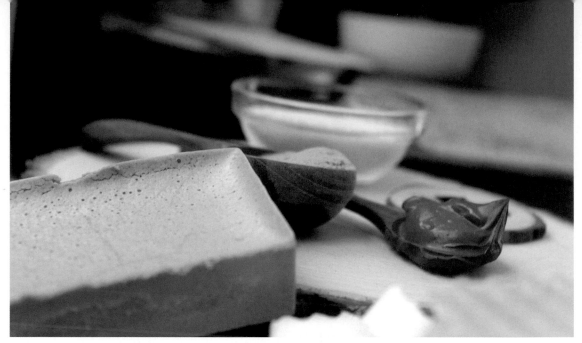

Dead Sea mud creates a lightweight bar full of nourishing minerals for both face and body.

WHIPPED MUD BAR FOR FACE AND BODY
FOR ALL SKIN TYPES ○ MAKES THREE 4-OUNCE (113G) BARS

With the magic of mineral-rich Dead Sea mud, this whipped bar brings the spa to the palm of your hand. Cleansing, gently extracting, and exfoliating, this powerful detox bar delivers a power-packed treatment to both face and body. Shea butter glycerin soap is blended with mud from the Dead Sea, sea salt, French green clay, spirulina, and marjoram and black spruce essential oils to make a beautiful sage-colored bar full of skin-loving nutrients and minerals. Like a mud bath, but much more pleasant, this is a deeply cleansing and restoring choice for both face and body.

EQUIPMENT
- Three 4-ounce (113g) soap molds (round, oval, rectangular, or shape of choosing)
- Kitchen scale
- Glass measuring cup
- Stir stick or spoon
- Smoothie blender
- Measuring spoons
- Wax paper

TIP: If you have any extra soap mix, pour it into paper cups to make mini travel bars!

INGREDIENTS
Base:
- 6 ounces (170g) clear glycerin soap blocks
- 2 ounces (56.5g) shea butter glycerin soap blocks

Additives:
- ⅛ teaspoon (0.5ml) spirulina
- 1½ teaspoons (7ml) Dead Sea mud
- 1½ teaspoons (7ml) French green clay
- 1½ teaspoons (7ml) sea salt

Essential Oils:
- 2 teaspoons (10ml) marjoram
- ½ teaspoon (2.5ml) black spruce

ALTERNATE ESSENTIAL OIL OPTIONS

For a refreshing and invigorating scent, use 1 teaspoon (5ml) peppermint.
For a sweet and light scent, use 1 tablespoon (15ml) pink grapefruit.

HOW TO MAKE

1. Weigh the clear and shea butter soap blocks and dice them into ½" (1.3cm) cubes. Add to a glass measuring cup and microwave in 1 minute increments, stirring in between with a wooden spoon or stir stick. Stop microwaving before it's entirely melted and stir until fully melted and still hot (don't allow to cool).

2. Pour into a smoothie blender and add the additives and essential oils. Blend for 5 to 10 seconds until the mixture is a uniform light sage color. Don't overblend as it can start to cool and become too thick to pour. You want the mixture to remain hot and liquid until poured into the soap molds.

3. Pour into the soap molds and allow to cool for 2 to 4 hours. To demold, place in the freezer for 20 minutes and then pop out of the molds onto wax paper or a cutting board.

HOW TO USE

Use daily or weekly on your face or body as desired. **Note:** Be sure to store on a soap dish and allow to fully dry between each use, as the mud makes this bar very water-soluble.

Spirulina is a type of microalgae that offers healing, gentle exfoliation, and a beautiful natural color.

A blend of clear and shea butter glycerin creates the base for this "spa in the palm of your hand."

Sea salt offers gentle cleansing and exfoliation with minerals to nurture the skin.

Cleansing, antimicrobial, healing mud from the Dead Sea has a high mineral and salt content.

French green clay offers natural extraction and cleansing.

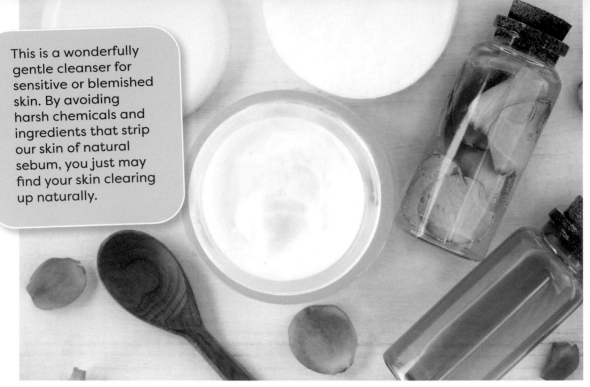

This is a wonderfully gentle cleanser for sensitive or blemished skin. By avoiding harsh chemicals and ingredients that strip our skin of natural sebum, you just may find your skin clearing up naturally.

This cold cream–style cleanser is filled with cleansing ingredients that won't dry out your skin.

ROSE TEA CREAM CLEANSER
FOR ALL SKIN TYPES ○ MAKES 12 OUNCES (350ML)

When you want to cleanse gently, rely on the healing and hydrating properties of tea seed oil, aloe vera, and jojoba. This light and lovely cold cream–style cleanser feels delightful on the skin and washes away makeup, dirt, and oil without drying your skin. This cleanser also features camellia tea seed oil, which is full of vitamins A, C, D, and E, lending antioxidant properties that protect against the free radicals that prematurely age our skin. *See Emulsion Tips on page 67.*

EQUIPMENT
- Small glass bowl
- Stirring spoon
- Thermometer, optional
- Glass measuring cup
- Measuring spoons
- Smoothie blender
- Glass jars
- Double boiler, optional

INGREDIENTS
Water Phase:
- 8 ounces (250ml) rose hydrosol
- 1 tablespoon (15ml) aloe vera gel
- 1 teaspoon (5ml) glycerin
- 1 teaspoon (5ml) citric acid

Oil Phase:
- 1 tablespoon (15ml) camellia tea seed oil
- 1 tablespoon (15ml) jojoba
- 3 tablespoons (21g) e-wax
- 1 teaspoon (5ml) stearic acid
- 5 drops vitamin E oil

Preservative:
- ½ teaspoon (2.5ml) Germaben II

HOW TO MAKE

Prepare the Water Phase

1. Combine water phase ingredients in a glass bowl and heat in the microwave for 1 minute until the citric acid is dissolved.
2. Stir and test the temperature with your thermometer. If it's not yet at 160°F–170°F (71°–77°C), microwave for 1 more minute and then set it aside.

Prepare the Oil Phase

1. Melt all the oil phase ingredients in a double boiler (or in the microwave, 1 minute at a time, stirring in between). Stir until all the butters are melted.
2. Heat to the same temperature as the water phase, letting cool if needed to reach the correct temperature range.

Blend the Phases

1. When phases are within the correct temperature range and are approximately the same temperature, pour the water phase into the small blender.
2. Add the oil phase—it should immediately turn white.
3. Blend for 5 to 10 seconds until fully combined.
4. Open the blender and allow the mixture to cool to 140°F (60°C). A temperature above that can compromise the preservative.
5. Add the preservative and blend for 5 to 10 seconds more.
6. Pour or spoon the mixture into glass jars and allow it to cool and thicken before capping them. Note: If it's hot out, put the open jars into the refrigerator to help the cream set. This is especially beneficial for lighter emulsions.

HOW TO USE

Massage into your face each morning and night, or whenever gentle cleaning is desired. Rinse with warm water and pat dry. Follow with toner and hydration if that's your preference, but I recommend first using only this cream and seeing how your skin feels. Mine is usually clear and perfectly happy using this as a daily cleanser without adding anything else afterward!

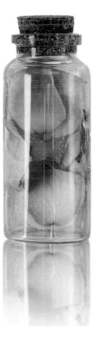

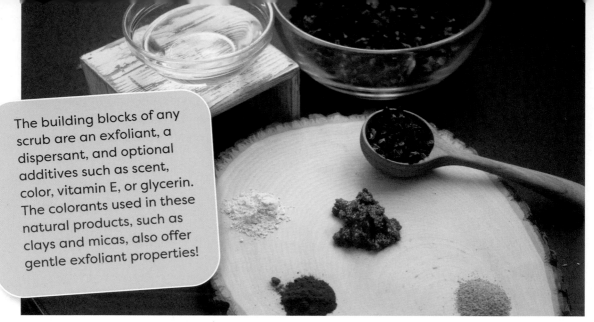

The building blocks of any scrub are an exfoliant, a dispersant, and optional additives such as scent, color, vitamin E, or glycerin. The colorants used in these natural products, such as clays and micas, also offer gentle exfoliant properties!

This decadent face scrub uses only natural botanicals, bypassing the microbeads used in most commercial brands, to leave your skin clear and radiant.

CHERRY ROSE FACE SCRUB

FOR ALL SKIN TYPES ○ MAKES THREE 2-OUNCE (60ML) JARS

Luxuriate in cherries and roses while giving your skin a triple gift of cleansing, exfoliation, and hydration. This beautiful scrub gives a deeply rejuvenating cleanse, sloughing away dead skin with the natural micro abrasion of powdered oats, cherry seeds, and rose petals, and hydrating with an ambrosia of fruity oils. It will quickly become an indulgent staple of your face-care routine once you see the difference it makes!

EQUIPMENT
- Mixing bowl
- Stirring spoon
- Measuring spoons
- Three 2-ounce (60ml) jars with lids

INGREDIENTS
Exfoliants:
- 1¼ cup (312ml) oatmeal powder
- ¼ cup (60ml) powdered cherry seeds
- 2 teaspoons (10ml) beetroot powder
- 2 teaspoons (10ml) powdered rose petals

Dispersants:
- ¼ cup (60ml) rose-infused jojoba
- 1 tablespoon (15ml) rose hip seed oil
- 1 tablespoon (15ml) pomegranate seed oil

- 1 tablespoon (15ml) cherry kernel oil
- 1 tablespoon (15ml) avocado oil
- 1 teaspoon (5ml) strawberry seed oil
- 1 teaspoon (5ml) vitamin E oil

Additives:
- 1 teaspoon (5ml) glycerin
- 24 drops grapefruit seed extract (GSE)

Essential Oil:
- 1 teaspoon (5ml) geranium rose

Preservative, optional in drier climates or if refrigerated:
- ½ teaspoon (2.5ml) Germaben II

DRY ALTERNATIVE

You can also make a dry version of this scrub that keeps indefinitely, doesn't risk mold, and exfoliates without carrier oils. Simply omit the dispersants and additives and mix as a dry powder. Then put a teaspoon of the powder in the palm of your hand and add a few drops of rose hydrosol or plain water to use.

HOW TO MAKE

1. Mix your dry ingredients in the mixing bowl until blended thoroughly.
2. Add your dispersants and additives and then mix until fully incorporated.
3. The scrub should feel like wet sand, with a tiny bit of excess oil on top (this will absorb over time).
4. Spoon into your jars and put on the lids.

HOW TO USE

Mix about 1 teaspoon (5ml) in the palm of your hand with a few drops of water. Gently massage your face, avoiding the area under your eyes. Rinse with warm water or wash off with the Rosewater Face Wash on page 72. Follow with toner and hydration, if desired.

Over time, your scrub will naturally dry a bit. Retexturize it as needed by adding more jojoba or avocado oil, or simply use it with more water.

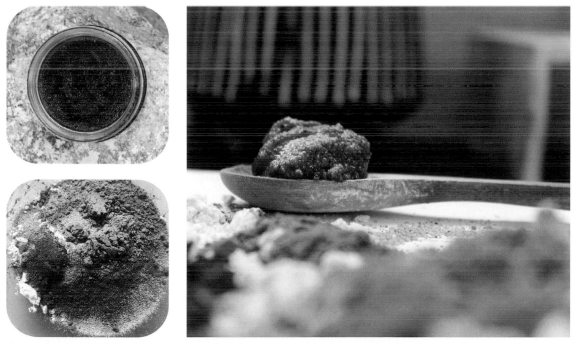

This scrub is beautiful and easy to make. The various ingredients blend into a soft and thorough exfoliant.

> Use scrubs either before or after washing. I prefer before, because then the cleansing step washes away everything the exfoliation stirred up!

Citrus is the star of the show in this scrub, but the clary sage essential oil provides skin-soothing benefits.

TANGERINE CLAY FACE SCRUB

FOR NORMAL TO OILY SKIN ○ MAKES 2 OUNCES (60ML)

This very fine face scrub feels like pure white sand and has the aroma of fresh tangerines. It offers gentle exfoliation for all skin types and the clary sage essential oil adds esters and monoterpenols that give this additional calming, anti-inflammatory properties.

EQUIPMENT

- Mixing bowl
- Stirring spoon
- Measuring spoons
- 2-ounce (60ml) jar with lid

INGREDIENTS

Exfoliant Base:
- 2 tablespoons (30ml) kaolin white clay
- 2 tablespoons (30ml) oat powder
- 2 teaspoons (10ml) orange peel powder
- 2 teaspoons (10ml) walnut shell powder

Dispersants and Additives:
- 2 tablespoons (30ml) calendula or sunflower oil
- 1 teaspoon (5ml) glycerin
- ¼ teaspoon (1.25ml) carrot seed oil
- ⅛ teaspoon (0.5ml) vitamin E oil
- 6 drops grapefruit seed extract (GSE), optional

Essential Oils:
- ⅛ teaspoon (0.5 ml) tangerine
- ⅛ teaspoon (0.5 ml) clary sage

DRY ALTERNATIVE

You can also make a dry version of this scrub that keeps indefinitely, doesn't risk mold, and exfoliates without carrier oils! Simply omit the dispersants and additives and mix as a dry powder. Then put a teaspoon of the powder in the palm of your hand and add a few drops of water to use.

HOW TO MAKE

1. Add dry ingredients to the mixing bowl and stir to incorporate.
2. Add the dispersants, additives, and essential oils, then stir thoroughly until fully incorporated. **Note:** Your scrub may appear to be a bit oily at first, but after sitting for a few hours, the ingredients will absorb the oil and the consistency will dry.
3. Spoon into the jar and put the lid on.

HOW TO USE

Massage into your face gently, avoiding the area under your eyes. Rinse with warm water and follow with a cleanser, toner, and hydration of your choice. If ever your scrub feels too dry, simply add more of your favorite carrier oil to restore it to your desired consistency.

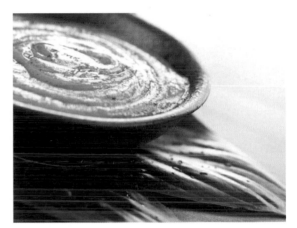

The natural powders in this exfoliant gently resurface your skin.

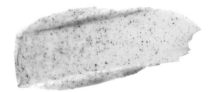

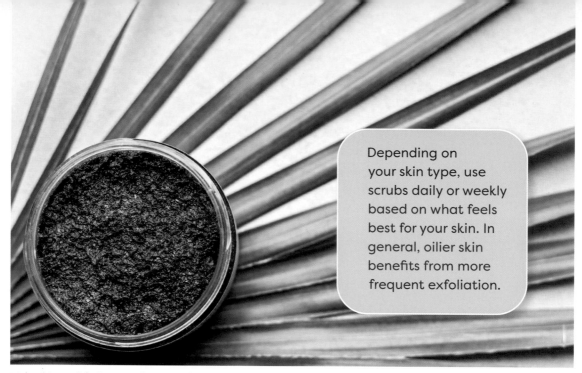

Depending on your skin type, use scrubs daily or weekly based on what feels best for your skin. In general, oilier skin benefits from more frequent exfoliation.

Make this scrub before you shower and use it right away to reveal hydrated, refreshed skin.

MANDARIN THYME CHIA SCRUB
FOR ALL SKIN TYPES ○ MAKES A SINGLE USE

This gel-like exfoliant is gentle, healing, plumping, and hydrating. Chia seeds are full of antioxidants that fight the free radical damage caused by UV exposure while soothing the skin. The two essential oils (mandarin and thyme) are monoterpenes, offering gentle antibacterial, anti-inflammatory, and antioxidant properties.

EQUIPMENT
- Small glass bowl
- Stirring spoon
- Measuring spoons
- Pipette

INGREDIENTS
Exfoliant Base:
- 1 tablespoon (15ml) chia seeds

Dispersant:
- 1 tablespoon (15ml) aloe vera gel

Essential Oils:
- 3–4 drops red mandarin
- 1 drop thyme linalol

HOW TO MAKE
1. Combine the chia seeds and aloe in the mixing bowl and stir to incorporate.
2. Drop in the essential oils and stir again.
3. Use immediately; this scrub does not keep.

HOW TO USE
Chia seeds can be a bit messy, so I recommend using this scrub in the shower. Spread it over your face and, if time allows, leave it on for 2 to 3 minutes before rinsing with warm water. Toss any excess; this scrub may only be used fresh as it will harden after sitting.

ROSEWATER FACE MIST

FOR ALL SKIN TYPES
MAKES 8 OUNCES (250ML)

Toners used with a cotton pad remove any last traces of dirt, grime, and impurities that remain on your face after washing and exfoliating, leaving your skin perfectly clean and ready for hydration. When used directly as a face spritz, they offer soothing hydration that is lighter than a lotion—a great way to refresh throughout the day, or after your morning cleanse.

EQUIPMENT
- Glass measuring cup
- Stir stick or spoon
- Glass spray bottles
- Measuring spoons

INGREDIENTS
- 4 ounces (125ml) rose hydrosol
- 4 ounces (125ml) witch hazel
- 1 teaspoon (5ml) glycerin
- 1 teaspoon (5ml) aloe vera

HOW TO MAKE
1. Add all ingredients to a glass measuring cup and stir.
2. Pour into glass spray bottles.

HOW TO USE
For gentle hydration, spritz onto a clean face. To tone and remove the final traces of dirt left after cleansing, spritz on your face and wipe with a cotton pad. Use any time to refresh and "wake up" your skin.

TIP: For an especially refreshing treat, store face mists in the refrigerator between uses.

TEA TREE BLEMISH REMEDY

FOR ALL SKIN TYPES
MAKES 1 OUNCE (30ML)

Many things can cause breakouts, such as stress and a poor diet. This remedy ensures that bacteria isn't the culprit by combining two heavy-hitting antibacterial essential oils to keep your skin perfectly clean and clear. Double or triple this recipe to fit whatever size spray bottle you'd like.

EQUIPMENT
- 1-ounce (30ml) glass spray bottle
- Pipette
- Small funnel
- Measuring spoons

INGREDIENTS
Base:
- 1 tablespoon (15ml) aloe vera gel
- 1 tablespoon (15ml) witch hazel

Essential Oils:
- 12 drops tea tree
- 4 drops rosemary

HOW TO MAKE
1. Using a funnel, add the aloe vera and witch hazel to the bottle.
2. Drop in the essential oils, cap the bottle, and shake to blend.

HOW TO USE
Apply a drop or two on blemishes or mist your face after washing to keep bacteria at bay.

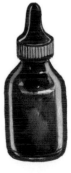

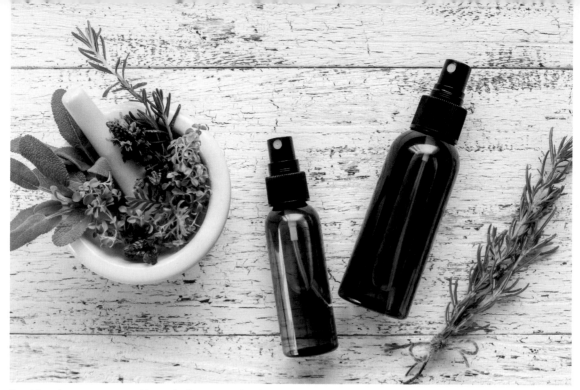

Soothing aloe, green tea, and lavender keep your skin fresh and vibrant.

LAVENDER ALOE TONER
FOR ALL SKIN TYPES ∘ MAKES 8 OUNCES (250ML)

A powerful antioxidant blend of lavender hydrosol and green tea, this lovely spray mixes the vitamins of green tea with the soothing and balancing esters and monoterpenols of lavender. Use it as a refreshing face mist or as a toner with a cotton pad.

EQUIPMENT
- 8-ounce (250ml) Glass measuring cup
- Measuring cup
- Wooden stir stick or stirring spoon
- Funnel
- Measuring spoons

INGREDIENTS
- 4 ounces (125ml) lavender hydrosol
- 4 ounces (125ml) brewed green tea
- 1 tablespoon (15ml) aloe vera

Preservative, optional if refrigerated:
- ⅛ teaspoon (0.5ml) Germaben II

HOW TO MAKE
1. Pour brewed, cooled green tea into the measuring cup.
2. Add the other ingredients and stir. Use the funnel to pour the mixture into the glass bottle.

HOW TO USE
For gentle hydration, spritz onto a clean face. To tone and remove the final traces of dirt left after cleansing, spritz on your face and wipe with a cotton pad. Use any time to refresh and "wake up" your skin. Leave refrigerated for best results, and use within a couple of months.

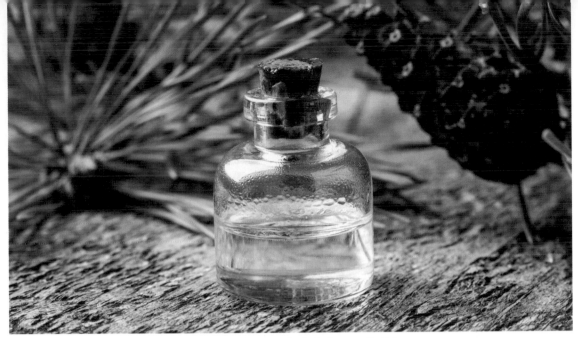

To calm, heal, and soften freshly shaven skin, use this natural splash that smells divine.

WHITE PINE AFTERSHAVE SPLASH
FOR ALL SKIN TYPES ○ MAKES 4 OUNCES (125ML)

Naturally soothe the skin after shaving with this refreshing aftershave splash. Look for organic, pure witch hazel, which naturally relieves irritation. The white pine essential oil smells fresh and invigorating, and has monoterpenes with soothing anti-inflammatory and analgesic properties.

EQUIPMENT
- Glass measuring cup
- Wooden stir stick or stirring spoon
- 4-ounce (125ml) bottle

INGREDIENTS
- 2 ounces (60ml) witch hazel
- 2 ounces (60ml) lavender hydrosol
- 1 teaspoon (5ml) glycerin
- 1 teaspoon (5ml) aloe vera gel

Essential Oils:
- ⅛ teaspoon (0.5 ml) white pine
- 3 drops lime or yuzu, optional

HOW TO MAKE
1. Add all ingredients to the measuring cup and stir.
2. Pour into the bottle.

HOW TO USE
Splash a teaspoon or so onto your face or on any skin that needs post-shave soothing.

ALTERNATIVES
Change up the scents—instead of lavender hydrosol, use distilled water or another floral or wood hydrosol (like chamomile, rose, or sandalwood).

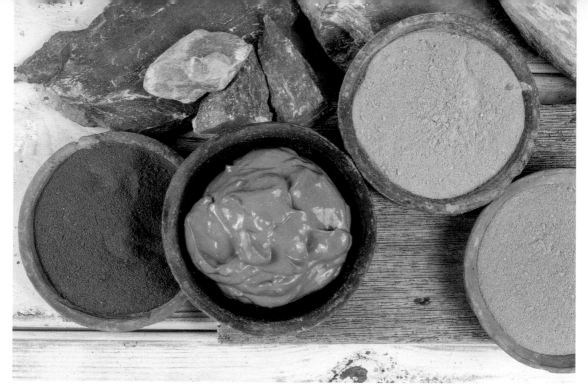

The minerals of the Dead Sea—in the form of salt and clay—blend beautifully with plant oils like argan, cherry kernel, and lavender to cleanse, tighten, and soften skin.

DEAD SEA MUD MASK

FOR NORMAL TO OILY SKIN ∘ MAKES 8 OUNCES (250ML)

This exquisitely cleansing, exfoliating, and extracting face mask restores and renews your skin, leaving it fresh, soft, and radiant. The Dead Sea's superpowers come from its minerals, including magnesium, calcium, bromide, potassium, and other trace elements that cleanse, nourish, and soften. Additionally, this mask is enhanced with jojoba, cherry kernel oil, argan oil, vitamin E, glycerin, white kaolin clay, and lavender and marjoram essential oils, which add additional antibacterial and skin-soothing properties, along with a lively scent.

EQUIPMENT

- Mixing bowl
- Measuring spoons
- Kitchen scale
- Glass jars

INGREDIENTS

Base:

- 8 ounces (226g) Dead Sea mud
- 1 tablespoon (15ml) white kaolin clay
- ½ teaspoon (2.5ml) jojoba
- ½ teaspoon (2.5ml) glycerin
- ¼ teaspoon (1.25ml) cherry kernel oil
- ¼ teaspoon (1.25ml) argan oil
- 4–6 drops vitamin E
- 4–6 drops grapefruit seed extract (GSE)

Essential Oils:

- ½ teaspoon (2.5ml) lavender
- ½ teaspoon (2.5ml) marjoram

HOW TO MAKE

1. Add all ingredients to the mixing bowl and stir until the texture is smooth and all the ingredients are incorporated.
2. Scoop into jars.

HOW TO USE

Massage over clean skin once a week or as desired. Leave on skin for 3 to 10 minutes, then rinse off with warm water. Follow with hydration or simply enjoy fresh, clean skin.

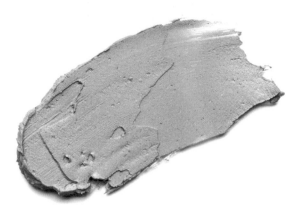

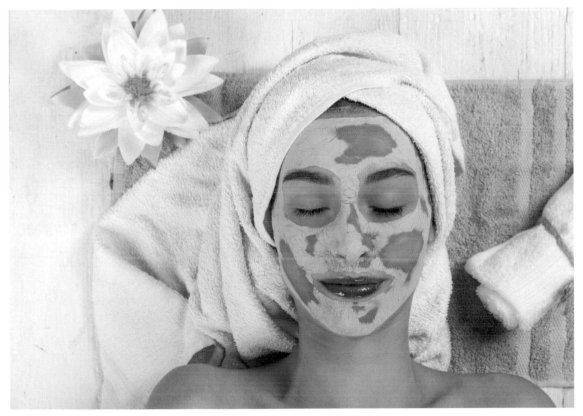

Incorporate this mask into your self-care routine and your skin will feel softened and rejuvenated.

SCENT ALTERNATIVES

Try making this mask by swapping the yuzu essential oil with other citruses, like lemon or lime. You'll create an equally refreshing option.

This mask uses healthy plant fats and antibacterial yuzu essential oil for a cleansing, clarifying facial treatment.

YUZU AVOCADO FACE MASK

FOR ALL SKIN TYPES ○ MAKES A SINGLE USE

Avocado offers natural exfoliation with antioxidants and minerals that remove dead skin cells, reduce inflammation, and hydrate the skin. Carrot seed oil is rich in beta carotene, vitamins A and E, and vitamin A, all of which balance and nourish the skin. Yuzu is an essential oil derived from the Japanese citrus fruit that is full of stimulating and antibacterial qualities and can counter the effects of free radicals. You won't want to rinse off this delicious-smelling mask!

EQUIPMENT

- Small glass bowl
- Measuring spoons
- Wooden stir stick or stirring spoon

INGREDIENTS

Base:
- ¼ of a medium avocado
- ¼ teaspoon (1.25ml) coconut oil (the fractionated, liquid form works well)
- ⅛ teaspoon (0.5 ml) carrot seed oil

Essential Oil:
- 6 drops yuzu

HOW TO MAKE

1. Mix all ingredients in a small bowl until soft and fully incorporated.

HOW TO USE

Spread over a clean face and allow to sit for 10 minutes as you relax. Rinse off with warm water and follow with a face mist or light hydration.

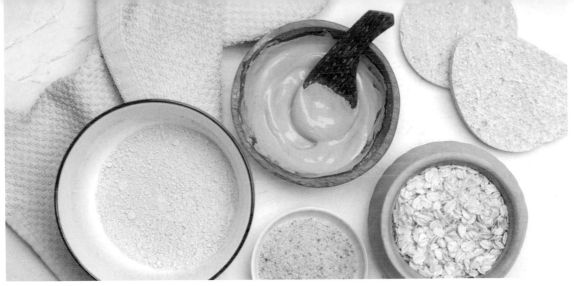

The kaolin white clay in this mask powerfully but gently extracts impurities from your skin.

CYPRESS CLAY MASK
FOR ALL SKIN TYPES ○ MAKES 2 OUNCES (60ML)

This gentle mask is extracting and clarifying, leaving your skin clean, soft, and hydrated. The clay is cleansing and exfoliating, sloughing off dirt, oil, and dead skin cells, while the coconut oil is antibacterial, and the glycerin moisturizes and seals in hydration. Calendula oil is soothing to the skin, full of anti-inflammatory and antimicrobial properties that can heal acne and restore skin elasticity. The two essential oils used here contain monoterpenes, which are also antibacterial and anti-inflammatory, adding to the healing nature of this mask. Ylang ylang has healing esters and sesquiterpenes that finish the mask off with a soothing, floral note.

EQUIPMENT
- Mixing bowl
- Measuring spoons
- Wooden stir stick or stirring spoon
- Small glass jar

INGREDIENTS
Exfoliants:
- 2 tablespoons (30ml) kaolin white clay
- 2 tablespoons (30ml) fine oat powder

Dispersants:
- 1 tablespoon (15ml) calendula oil
- 1 tablespoon (15ml) coconut oil
- 1 teaspoon (5ml) glycerin

Additives:
- ⅛ teaspoon (0.5ml) vitamin E oil
- 6 drops grapefruit seed extract (GSE)

Essential Oils:
- 8 drops cypress
- 4 drops bergamot
- 1 drop ylang ylang

HOW TO MAKE
1. If using solid coconut oil, soften it in the microwave for 5 seconds. If using fractionated, liquid coconut oil, skip to step 2.
2. Add all the ingredients to the mixing bowl and stir until thoroughly combined.
3. Transfer to a small glass jar.

HOW TO USE
Spread 1 to 2 teaspoons over a clean face and relax for 5–10 minutes or until the mask is dry. Rinse with warm water and apply a face mist or hydration of your choosing.

Adjust the amount of cardamom essential oil in this blend based on the strength of aroma you prefer.

CARDAMOM-ROSE WHIPPED CRÈME

FOR NORMAL TO DRY SKIN ○ MAKES 16 OUNCES (500ML)

This thick and fluffy whipped crème uses the pure essence of rose hydrosol and skin-soothing cardamom essential oil, plus strawberry seed oil, sunflower oil, and aloe vera, to create a deeply hydrating and creamy lotion. Use on your face, hands, or anywhere you crave delightfully soft and fluffy hydration and a light aroma. Homemade lotions are on a completely different level from anything you can buy in stores—whether you prefer milky and silky or thick and fluffy, you'll never want to use a waxy store-bought cream again! *See Emulsion Tips on page 67.*

EQUIPMENT

- Small glass bowl
- Glass measuring cup
- Thermometer, optional
- Measuring spoons
- Smoothie blender
- Glass jars
- Double boiler, optional

INGREDIENTS

Water Phase:
- 8 ounces (250ml) rose hydrosol
- 1 tablespoon (15ml) aloe vera gel
- 1 teaspoon (5ml) glycerin
- 1 teaspoon (5ml) citric acid

Oil Phase:
- ¾ teaspoon (3.75ml) fractionated coconut oil
- ½ tablespoon (7ml) strawberry seed oil
- ½ tablespoon (7ml) sunflower oil
- 3 tablespoons (45ml) rose-infused jojoba
- 3 tablespoons (21g) e-wax
- 1 teaspoon (5ml) stearic acid
- 6 drops vitamin E oil

Essential Oil:
- ⅛ teaspoon (0.5ml) cardamom (or a bit less for more delicate aroma)

Preservative:
- ¾ teaspoon (3.75ml) Germaben II

MOISTURIZER ESSENTIAL: PRESERVATIVE

Lotions are the one product where you don't want to skip the preservative—any product made with water can grow mold. At least 0.3 to 1 percent of the total weight of your lotions, scrubs, and other products made with water should be preservative. Add the preservative when your product temperature is 140°F (60°C) or lower, as higher temperatures can degrade the preservative's effectiveness.

HOW TO MAKE

Prepare the Water Phase

1. Combine water phase ingredients in a glass bowl and heat in the microwave for 1 minute until the citric acid is dissolved.
2. Stir and test the temperature with your thermometer. If it's not yet at 160°F–170°F (71°–77°C), microwave for 1 more minute and then set it aside.

Prepare the Oil Phase

1. Melt all the oil phase ingredients in a double boiler (or in the microwave, 1 minute at a time, stirring in between). Stir until all the butters are melted.
2. Heat to the same temperature as the water phase, letting cool if needed to reach the correct temperature range.

Blend the Phases

1. When phases are within the correct temperature range and are approximately the same temperature, pour the water phase into the small blender.
2. Add the oil phase—it should immediately turn white.
3. Blend for 5 to 10 seconds until fully combined.
4. Open the blender and allow the mixture to cool to 140°F (60°C). A temperature above that can compromise the preservative.
5. Add the essential oil and preservative, and blend for 5 to 10 seconds more.
6. Pour or spoon the mixture into glass jars and allow it to cool and thicken before capping them.

HOW TO USE

Massage into your face each morning and night, or whenever you need hydration. You can also use this lotion for your hands and body, as needed.

Rather than using rose essential oil—which, when authentic and pure, is priced like gold—this recipe uses rose-infused jojoba, which offers the same beautiful scent and healing benefits at a more affordable cost.

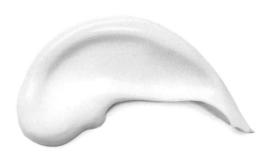

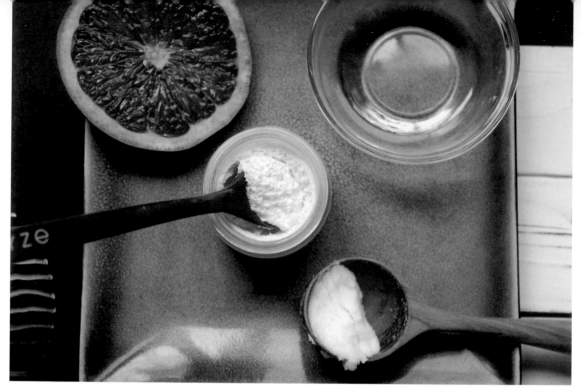

This light and fluffy face cream has the detoxifying qualities and heavenly aroma of fresh grapefruit.

GRAPEFRUIT LIGHT LOTION

FOR NORMAL TO OILY SKIN ○ MAKES 8 OUNCES (250ML)

This light and luscious lotion benefits from aloe vera, argan and sunflower oils, jojoba, and distilled water, creating a nonclogging, hydrating face or hand moisturizer. With the fresh and delicate aroma and detoxifying chemical properties of pink grapefruit essential oil, this light lotion absorbs quickly and helps clarify oily and combination skin, keeping it hydrated but never greasy. This fluffy cream is exquisitely refreshing and bright. *See Emulsion Tips on page 67.*

EQUIPMENT

- Small glass bowl
- Glass measuring cup
- Thermometer, optional
- Measuring spoons
- Smoothie blender
- Glass jars
- Double boiler, optional

INGREDIENTS

Water Phase:
- 8 ounces (250ml) distilled water
- 1 tablespoon (15ml) aloe vera gel
- ½ teaspoon (2.5ml) glycerin
- ½ teaspoon (2.5ml) citric acid

Oil Phase:
- 2 tablespoons (30ml) jojoba
- 1 teaspoon (5ml) coconut oil
- 1 teaspoon (5ml) argan oil
- 1 teaspoon (5ml) sunflower oil
- 4 teaspoons (16g) e-wax
- 1 teaspoon (5ml) stearic acid
- 6 drops vitamin E oil

Essential Oil:
- 1 tablespoon (15ml) pink grapefruit

Preservative:
- ¾ teaspoon (3.75ml) Germaben II

HOW TO MAKE

Prepare the Water Phase

1. Combine water phase ingredients in a glass bowl and heat in the microwave for 1 minute until the citric acid is dissolved.
2. Stir and test the temperature with your thermometer. If it's not yet at 160°F–170°F (71°–77°C), microwave for 1 more minute and then set it aside.

Prepare the Oil Phase

1. Melt all the oil phase ingredients in a double boiler (or in the microwave, 1 minute at a time, stirring in between). Stir until all the butters are melted.
2. Heat to the same temperature as the water phase, letting cool if needed to reach the correct temperature range.

Blend the Phases

1. When phases are within the correct temperature range and are approximately the same temperature, pour the water phase into the small blender.
2. Add the oil phase—it should immediately turn white.
3. Blend for 5 to 10 seconds until fully combined.

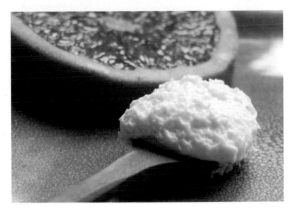

Coconut oil, argan, and aloe vera create a luscious, whipped texture.

4. Open the blender and allow the mixture to cool to 140°F (60°C). A temperature above that can compromise the preservative.
5. Add the essential oil and preservative, and blend for 5 to 10 seconds more.
6. Pour or spoon the mixture into glass jars and allow it to cool and thicken before capping them.

HOW TO USE

Massage into your face or anywhere you crave fresh, light hydration.

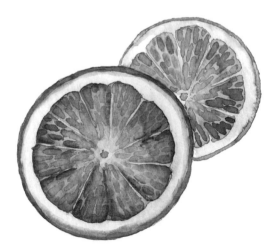

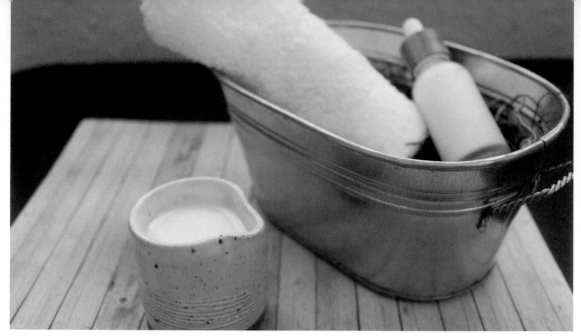

This face milk is easily absorbed and full of skin-loving nutrients. Its healthy fats smooth skin cells and help maintain skin's elasticity, in a lightweight formulation that won't clog pores.

COCONUT FACE MILK
FOR NORMAL TO OILY SKIN ○ MAKES 12 OUNCES (355ML)

This light and lovely face milk offers beautiful hydration for all skin types, leaving your face soft, fresh, and hydrated. This powerhouse blends nutrient-rich coconut milk (high in vitamin C, which helps maintain elasticity, clarity, and brightness), aloe vera, and carrot seed oil (which has vitamin A and antibacterial and antioxidant qualities), with the sweet, heavenly mix of jasmine and orange scents. *See Emulsion Tips on page 67.*

EQUIPMENT
- Small glass bowl
- Glass measuring cup
- Thermometer, optional
- Measuring spoons
- Smoothie blender
- Glass jars
- Double boiler, optional

INGREDIENTS
Water Phase:
- 2 ounces (60ml) low-fat coconut milk
- 6 ounces (175ml) distilled water
- 1 tablespoon (15ml) aloe vera gel
- ¾ teaspoon (3.75 ml) glycerin
- ¾ teaspoon (3.75 ml) citric acid

Oil Phase:
- ¾ teaspoon (3.75 ml) fractionated coconut oil
- ½ teaspoon (2.5 ml) carrot seed oil
- ½ teaspoon (2.5 ml) argan oil
- 1 tablespoon (15 ml) sunflower oil
- 1 teaspoon (3g) e-wax
- ¾ teaspoon (3.75 ml) stearic acid
- 6 drops vitamin E oil

Essential Oils:
- 1½ teaspoons (7ml) orange
- ½ teaspoons (2.5ml) jasmine

Preservative:
- ¾ teaspoon (3.75ml) Germaben II

HOW TO MAKE

Prepare the Water Phase

1. Combine water phase ingredients in a glass bowl and heat in the microwave for 1 minute until the citric acid is dissolved.
2. Stir and test the temperature with your thermometer. If it's not yet at 160°F–170°F (71°–77°C), microwave for 1 more minute and then set it aside.

Prepare the Oil Phase

1. Melt all the oil phase ingredients in a double boiler (or in the microwave, 1 minute at a time, stirring in between). Stir until all the butters are melted.
2. Heat to the same temperature as the water phase, letting cool if needed to reach the correct temperature range.

Blend the Phases

1. When phases are within the correct temperature range and are approximately the same temperature, pour the water phase into the small blender.
2. Add the oil phase—it should immediately turn white.
3. Blend for 5 to 10 seconds until fully combined.
4. Open the blender and allow the mixture to cool to 140°F (60°C). A temperature above that can compromise the preservative.
5. Add the essential oils and preservative, and blend for 5 to 10 seconds more.
6. Pour or spoon the mixture into glass jars and allow it to cool and thicken in the refrigerator before capping them.

HOW TO USE

Because very little e-wax is used to create this product's milky consistency, give your face milk a good shake to reincorporate before each use. Pour the desired amount into your hands and massage over a clean and toned face.

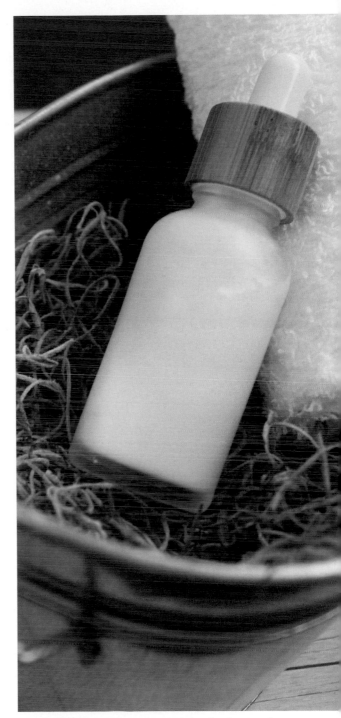

I like to package my face milk in little bottles, leaving them refrigerated until ready to use.

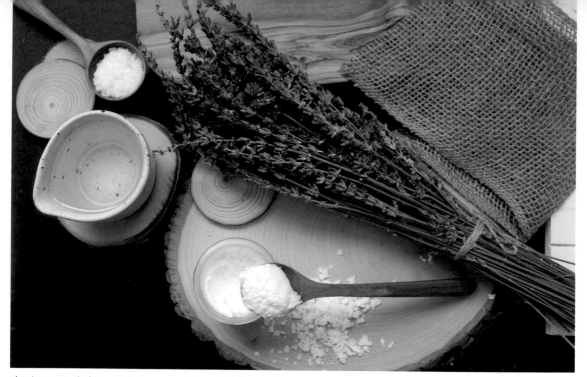

This lotion's oil phase includes mango butter, jojoba, and coconut oil to create a thick, rich crème that's great for regular use on your face, hands, and feet, or under your eyes at bedtime.

LAVENDER WHIPPED CRÈME

FOR NORMAL TO DRY SKIN, OR ALL SKIN TYPES IF USED UNDER EYES OR ON BODY
MAKES 8 OUNCES (250ML)

This thick and luscious moisturizer can be used on your face, hands, feet, or really anywhere you need soothing hydration. The mango butter offers natural sun protection, the aloe and oils soothe and hydrate, and the lavender essential oil delivers the heavenly aroma of lavender fields to your skin. *See Emulsion Tips on page 67.*

EQUIPMENT
- Small glass bowl
- Glass measuring cup
- Thermometer, optional
- Measuring spoons
- Smoothie blender
- Glass bottles with caps or dropper tops
- Double boiler, optional

INGREDIENTS
Water Phase:
- ½ cup (125ml) lavender hydrosol or distilled water
- ¼ cup (60ml) aloe vera gel
- 1½ teaspoons (7ml) glycerin
- ⅛ teaspoon (0.5ml) citric acid

Oil Phase:
- 2 tablespoons (30ml) mango butter
- 1 tablespoon (15ml) coconut oil
- 1 tablespoon (15ml) avocado oil
- 2 teaspoons (10ml) jojoba
- 3 tablespoons (21g) e-wax
- ⅛ teaspoon (0.5ml) stearic acid

Essential Oil:
- 1½ teaspoons (7ml) lavender

Preservative:
- ½ teaspoon (2.5ml) Germaben II

HOW TO MAKE

Prepare the Water Phase

1. Combine water phase ingredients in a glass bowl and heat in the microwave for 1 minute until the citric acid is dissolved.
2. Stir and test the temperature with your thermometer. If it's not yet at 160°F–170°F (71°–77°C), microwave for 1 more minute and then set it aside.

Prepare the Oil Phase

1. Melt all the oil phase ingredients in a double boiler (or in the microwave, 1 minute at a time, stirring in between). Stir until all the butters are melted.
2. Heat to the same temperature as the water phase, letting cool if needed to reach the correct temperature range.

Blend the Phases

1. When phases are within the correct temperature range and are approximately the same temperature, pour the water phase into the small blender.
2. Add the oil phase—it should immediately turn white.
3. Blend for 5 to 10 seconds until fully combined.
4. Open the blender and allow the mixture to cool to 140°F (60°C). A temperature above that can compromise the preservative.
5. Add the essential oil and preservative, and blend for 5 to 10 seconds more.
6. Pour the mixture into glass bottles.

HOW TO USE

Massage into your cleaned, exfoliated face or anywhere you crave hydration. Dab under your eyes at bedtime to take advantage of lavender's sedative properties.

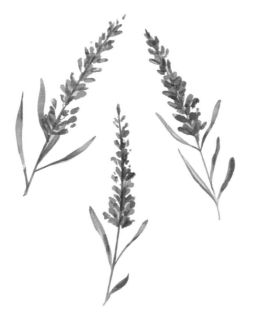

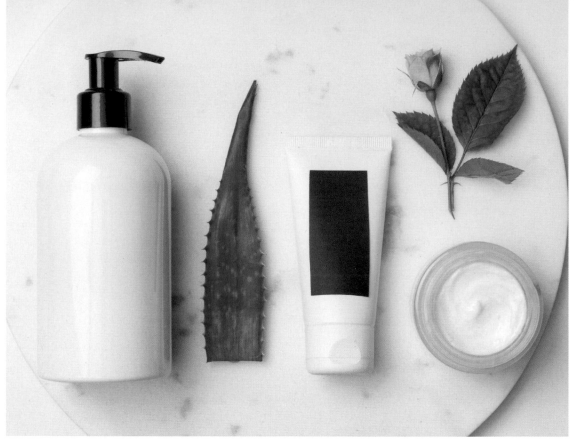

This thick cream moisturizes and protects your most delicate skin by combining skin-healing ingredients.

ROSE UNDER-EYE CREAM

FOR ALL SKIN TYPES ○ MAKES 8 OUNCES (250ML)

This thick whipped cream keeps the delicate skin under your eyes hydrated and protected from excess sun, aging, and dark circles. Coconut oil offers anti-inflammatory qualities and jojoba is a natural moisturizer, keeping your eyes feeling fresh and vibrant. *See Emulsion Tips on page 67.*

EQUIPMENT

- Small glass bowl
- Glass measuring cup
- Thermometer, optional
- Smoothie blender
- Measuring spoons
- Glass jars
- Double boiler, optional

INGREDIENTS

Water Phase:
- ½ cup (125ml) rose hydrosol
- 1 tablespoon (15ml) aloe vera gel
- 1 teaspoon (5ml) glycerin
- ½ teaspoon (2.5ml) citric acid

Oil Phase:
- 1 teaspoon (5ml) fractionated coconut oil

- 1 tablespoon (15ml) sunflower oil
- 1 tablespoon (15ml) jojoba
- 2 tablespoons (14g) e-wax
- 2 teaspoons (10ml) stearic acid
- 3 drops vitamin E oil

Preservative:
- ½ teaspoon (2.5ml) Germaben II

Since this recipe makes a large quantity of eye cream, try pouring it into several small containers and keeping them in the refrigerator until ready to use or spread the love and give them to friends and loved ones! You can also use it as an allover face or décolletage cream.

HOW TO MAKE

Prepare the Water Phase

1. Combine water phase ingredients in a glass bowl and heat in the microwave for 1 minute until the citric acid is dissolved.
2. Stir and test the temperature with your thermometer. If it's not yet at 160°F–170°F (71°–77°C), microwave for 1 more minute and then set it aside.

Prepare the Oil Phase

1. Melt all the oil phase ingredients in a double boiler (or in the microwave, 1 minute at a time, stirring in between). Stir until all the butters are melted.
2. Heat to the same temperature as the water phase, letting cool if needed to reach the correct temperature range.

Blend the Phases

1. When phases are within the correct temperature range and are approximately the same temperature, pour the water phase into the small blender.
2. Add the oil phase—it should immediately turn white.
3. Blend for 5 to 10 seconds until fully combined.
4. Open the blender and allow the mixture to cool to 140°F (60°C). A temperature above that can compromise the preservative.

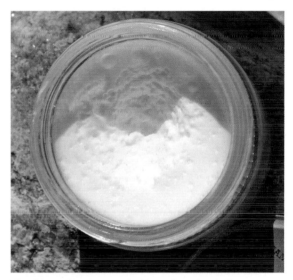

The skin under your eyes is thin and can be easily damaged. Protect and soothe it with this creamy treat!

5. Add the preservative and blend for 5 to 10 seconds more.
6. Pour or spoon the mixture into glass jars and allow it to cool and thicken before capping them.

HOW TO USE

Dab under your eyes to soften and protect the delicate skin. Use before applying makeup, at bedtime, or anytime you want to hydrate and restore this area.

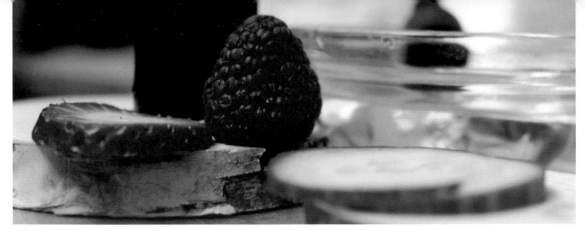

Plant the seeds of radiant skin with this luscious elixir that blends oils known for their antiaging, antioxidant, and anti-inflammatory properties.

RADIANCE SEED SERUM
FOR ALL SKIN TYPES ○ MAKES 1 OUNCE (30ML)

This regenerating serum helps restore, renew, and rejuvenate your skin, leaving a vibrant complexion because of its nourishing plant collagens, essential amino acids, vitamins, minerals, and precious phytosqualane. Use just a few drops nightly and wake up with clear, radiant skin. If you don't have all ten oils, you can substitute with similar oils you do have to create an equally lovely restoring serum. You may just want to double the recipe and keep a second bottle in the refrigerator so you never run out!

EQUIPMENT
- Glass measuring cup
- Mixing bowl
- Wooden stir stick or stirring spoon
- Measuring spoons
- 1-ounce (30ml) dark glass dropper bottle

INGREDIENTS
Base:
- 1 teaspoon (5ml) jojoba
- 1 teaspoon (5ml) avocado oil
- ½ teaspoon (2.5ml) cucumber seed oil
- ½ teaspoon (2.5ml) argan oil
- ½ teaspoon (2.5ml) rose hip seed oil
- ½ teaspoon (2.5ml) camellia tea seed oil
- ½ teaspoon (2.5ml) strawberry seed oil
- ½ teaspoon (2.5ml) red raspberry seed oil
- ½ teaspoon (2.5ml) pomegranate seed oil
- ½ teaspoon (2.5ml) watermelon seed oil
- ½ teaspoon (2.5ml) cherry seed oil

Additives:
- 12 drops vitamin E
- 12 drops grapefruit seed extract (GSE)

Essential Oils:
- ¼ teaspoon (1.25ml) geranium rose
- 6 drops balsam copaiba, optional

HOW TO MAKE
1. Add all the base ingredients, additives, and essential oils to the mixing bowl. Stir to combine.
2. Pour into the dark dropper bottle (the dark color helps protects the oils from going rancid). Cap.

HOW TO USE
After exfoliating, cleansing, and toning, place 5 to 6 drops into the palms of your hands, rub together, and then massage into the skin of the face, including under the eyes. Wake up to clear, radiant skin!

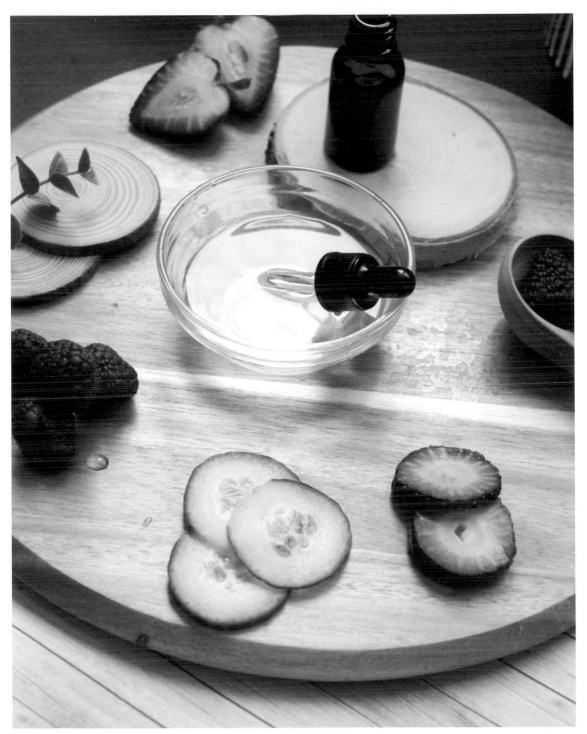

Oils compressed from fruit seeds are full of antioxidants, vitamins, and essential fatty acids, and your face will love them.

Butters, lotions, powders, and waxes all combine beautifully
to create luxurious bases for your essential oil creations.

BODY CARE RECIPES

Natural products help us clean, soothe, heal, and protect just as well as commercial products, but without the harmful chemicals and unnecessary excess packaging. We can keep our teeth clean and polished, our skin soft and hydrated, and our breath and bodies fresh by tapping into the healing properties and beautiful aromas of essential oils. Next time you need anything for your skin, hair, or body, check these recipes first to see what you can whip up with the items in your cupboard. Your body will delight in their healthy, wholesome properties.

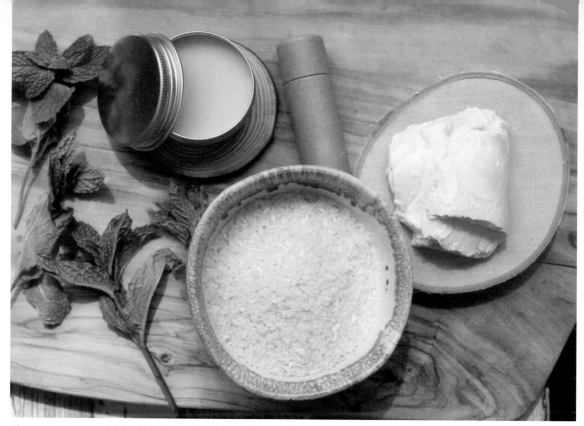

The sweet secret to this lip balm is unrefined cocoa butter, which smells exactly like chocolate.

CHOCOLATE MINT LIP BALM

MAKES EIGHT OVERSIZED ⅓-OUNCE (9ML) LIP BALM TUBES OR SIXTEEN STANDARD
³⁄₁₆-OUNCE (5.5ML) LIP BALM TUBES OR FIVE 1-OUNCE (30ML) METAL TINS

The combined chocolate essence of pure cocoa butter and peppermint essential oil creates a decadent chocolate mint moisturizer for your lips, while offering natural sun protection. It smells so good you'll want to eat it!

EQUIPMENT

- Lip balm tubes or tins
- Glass bowl
- Measuring spoons
- Large pipette
- Wooden stir stick
- Double boiler, optional

INGREDIENTS

Base:

- 1½ teaspoons (7.5g) unrefined cocoa butter
- 4 tablespoons (22g) candelilla wax
- 2 tablespoons (30ml) coconut oil
- 2 tablespoons (30ml) avocado oil
- 1 tablespoon (15ml) jojoba
- 12 drops Vitamin E oil, optional

Essential Oil:

- ½ teaspoon (2.5ml) peppermint

HOW TO MAKE

1. Melt your cocoa butter, wax, and coconut oil in a small glass bowl either over a double boiler or in the microwave, 15 seconds at a time, stopping to stir in between with the wooden stir stick.

2. Once fully melted, add the avocado oil, jojoba, vitamin E (if desired) and essential oil. Stir to blend.

3. Using your pipette, carefully fill each tube, slowing as you reach the top so you can fill just enough to create a slight mound of liquid at the top. Work quickly while the liquid is hot. (If the liquid starts to cool, reheat it. You may need a fresh pipette if the wax dries.) If using tins, pour slowly into each. There is usually a stopping line about ⅛" from the top.

4. Leave uncapped for 30 minutes or until fully solidified before capping and labeling.

HOW TO USE

Apply to your lips as needed to keep them soft, hydrated, and protected from the sun.

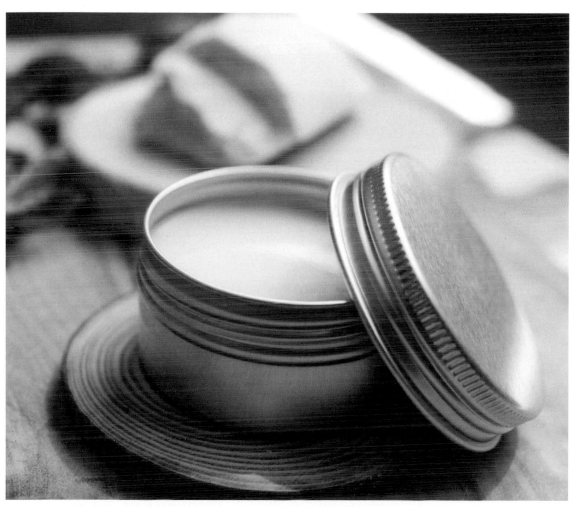

Capture your balm in tins or tubes, depending on your preferred application method.

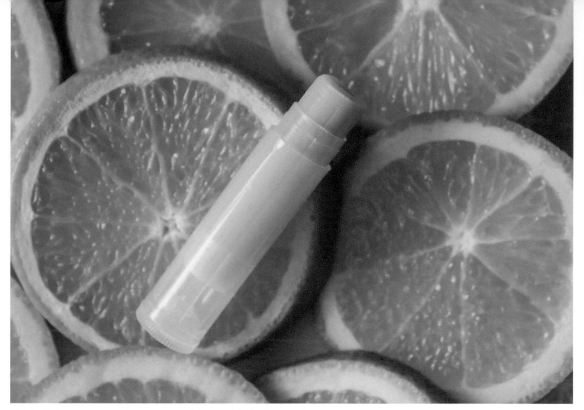

This lip balm is sweet and creamy, an addictive delight for your lips.

ORANGE CRUSH LIP BALM

MAKES EIGHT OVERSIZED ⅓-OUNCE (9ML) LIP BALM TUBES OR SIXTEEN STANDARD
³⁄₁₆-OUNCE (5.5ML) LIP BALM TUBES OR FIVE 1-OUNCE (30ML) METAL TINS

This sweet treat combines orange essential oil and vanilla absolute to create an aroma reminiscent of
Orange Crush® soda and soothing protection that delights every time you apply it. Sweet and creamy, this
balm keeps your lips hydrated and healthy.

EQUIPMENT

- Lip balm tubes or tins
- Glass bowl
- Measuring spoons
- Large pipette
- Wooden stir stick or stirring spoon
- Double boiler, optional

INGREDIENTS

Base:

- 2 teaspoons (10ml) mango butter
- 4 tablespoons (22g) candelilla wax
- 1 tablespoon (15ml) jojoba
- 2 tablespoons (30ml) coconut oil
- 2 tablespoons (30ml) olive oil
- 12 drops vitamin E oil, optional

Essential Oils:

- ¼ teaspoon (1.25ml) vanilla absolute
- 1 tablespoon (15ml) sweet orange

HOW TO MAKE

1. Melt the mango butter, wax, and coconut oil in a small glass bowl either over a double boiler or in the microwave, 15 seconds at a time, stopping to stir.
2. Once fully melted, add the olive oil, jojoba, vitamin E (if desired), and essential oils. Stir to blend.
3. Using your pipette, carefully fill each tube, slowing as you reach the top so you can fill just enough to create a slight mound of liquid at the top. Work quickly while the liquid is hot. (If the liquid starts to cool, reheat it. You may need a fresh pipette if the wax dries.) If using tins, pour slowly into each. There is usually a stopping line about ⅛" from the top.
4. Leave uncapped for 30 minutes or until fully solidified before capping and labeling.

HOW TO USE

Apply to your lips as needed to keep them soft and hydrated.

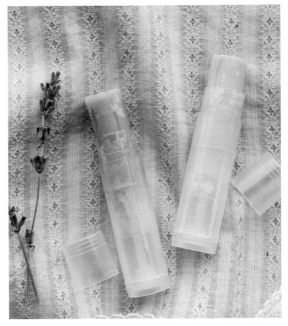

Homemade lip balms make a useful and crowd-pleasing gift any time of year.

TIP: To enhance the vanilla essence, try substituting plain jojoba for vanilla-infused jojoba.

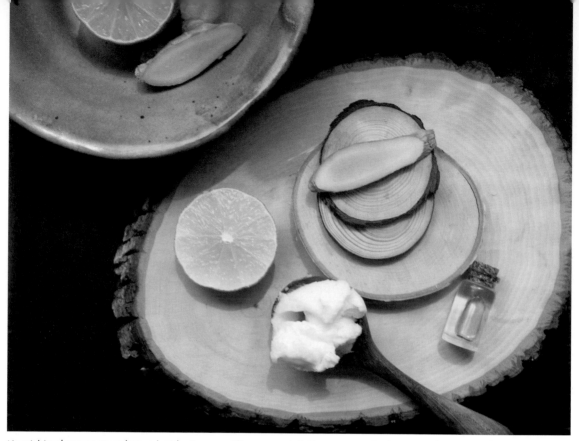

Nourishing butters are enhanced with ginger and lime essential oils to create a hydrating and protective body butter.

GINGER LIME WHIPPED BODY BUTTER

MAKES 2 ½–3 CUPS (625–750ML) WHIPPED BUTTER

Whipped plant butter is a rich treat for your skin that's made even better with the classic culinary combination of lime and ginger essential oils, softening and hydrating wherever you need it most. This thick, creamy butter offers a light natural SPF and is a rich remedy for even the driest skin.

EQUIPMENT

- Mixing bowl
- Electric mixer
- Measuring cups
- Measuring spoons
- Glass jars or metal tins
- Double boiler, optional

INGREDIENTS

Base:

- 1 cup (250ml) shea butter
- ½ cup (125ml) coconut oil
- ½ cup (125ml) almond oil

Essential Oils:

- 1 tablespoon (15ml) lime
- 1 teaspoon (5ml) ginger

HOW TO MAKE

1. Melt shea butter and coconut oil in the top of a double boiler or in the microwave in 30 second increments, stopping to stir.
2. Once fully melted, let sit for 15 minutes to temper (and prevent later crystallization, which can happen when using shea butter).
3. Stir in the almond oil and essential oils until they are fully incorporated. Blend the mix with your electric mixer for a few seconds and then place it in the freezer.
4. Check the mix after 15 minutes—the mixture at the edges of the bowl should start to harden and lighten in color. Take it out and stir to incorporate the harder parts at the edges into the rest of the mix.
5. Whip the mix with your electric mixer until it reaches a uniform consistency. Return it to the freezer.
6. Repeat steps 4 and 5 two more times or until the mixture is solid but soft enough to scoop.
7. Use a spoon to transfer the butter to glass jars or metal tins. Cap.

HOW TO USE

Massage into the skin after showering or anytime you crave deep hydration.

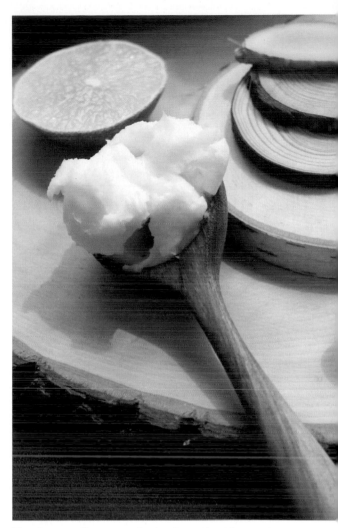

Plant butters offer a protective barrier on the skin, creating natural, gentle sun protection.

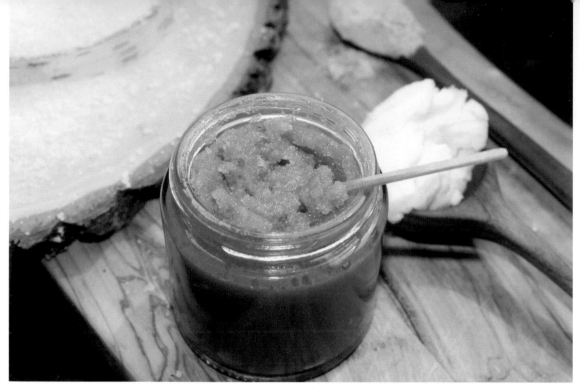

Naturally colored with clay, sugar scrubs make beautiful gifts for yourself and those you love.

PINK BLISS SCRUB

MAKES 16 OUNCES (500ML)

Luxuriate in this deeply moisturizing and gently exfoliating body scrub that sloughs away dead skin and leaves behind soft, hydrated skin. The essential oils are uplifting, while the sugar offers a softening gentler exfoliation than salt, with a natural source of glycolic acid that breaks down layers of dead skin and smooths its surface.

EQUIPMENT

- Large mixing bowl
- Glass measuring cup
- Kitchen scale
- Stirring spoon
- Glass jars

INGREDIENTS

Exfoliants:
- 16 ounces (500ml) organic white sugar
- 1 tablespoon (15ml) pink clay

Dispersants:
- 2 ounces (56g) shea butter
- 2 ounces (56g) coconut oil
- 3 ounces (85g) sunflower oil
- 1 tablespoon (15ml) jojoba
- 1 tablespoon (15ml) vegetable glycerin

- 6 drops grapefruit seed extract (GSE), optional
- 6 drops vitamin E oil, optional

Essential Oils:
- 2 teaspoons (10ml) pink grapefruit
- 1 teaspoon (5ml) sweet orange
- ⅛ teaspoon (0.5ml) yuzu

HOW TO MAKE

1. Stir the pink clay into the sugar until it's a uniform pale pink color throughout.
2. Melt the coconut oil and shea butter in the microwave for 30 seconds. Stir and microwave a few more seconds if needed to fully liquefy.
3. Add the melted oil and butter to the sugar and stir.
4. Add the essential oils and mix until fully integrated. The liquid should feel like wet sand—add a bit more sunflower oil or sugar if needed to create your desired consistency.
5. Scoop into the jars and cap.

HOW TO USE

After cleansing in the shower, massage this scrub all over your body and rinse. Your skin is now soft, exfoliated, and hydrated—no need for lotion.

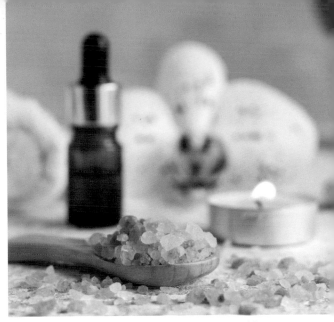

My recipe uses white sugar to exfoliate, but you could change the texture by using pink salt instead.

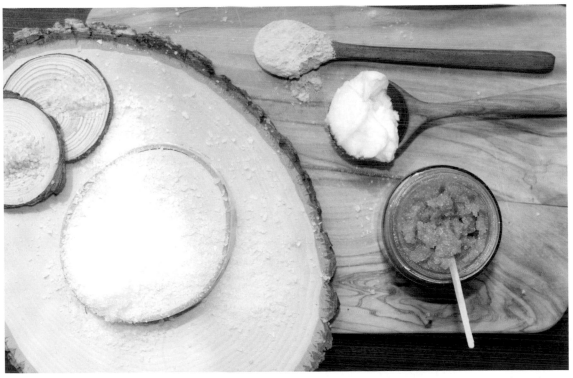

The beautiful blend of butters, clay, and oil with sugar creates a luxurious treat for the body that is easy to make and delightful to use.

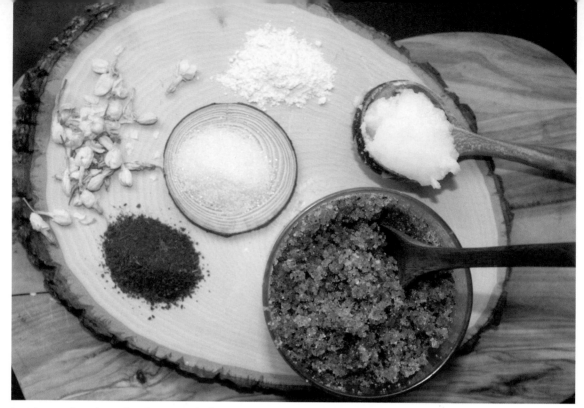

Jasmine petals and powdered coconut shells create an exotic, nurturing body scrub.

JASMINE COCONUT SCRUB
MAKES 8 OUNCES (250 ML)

The rich, tropical aroma of jasmine essential oil is seductive and soothing. It's used here in conjunction with dried jasmine petals to make a gently exfoliating and skin-loving treat that whisks cares away.

EQUIPMENT

- Mixing bowl
- Wooden stir stick or stirring spoon
- Glass jars
- Mortar and pestle or coffee grinder, optional

INGREDIENTS

Exfoliant Base:

- 1 cup (250ml) organic white sugar
- ¼ cup (125ml) coconut oil
- 1 tablespoon (15ml) white clay
- 1 tablespoon (15ml) dried jasmine petals
- 1 tablespoon (15ml) powdered coconut shells

Dispersant:

- ⅓ cup (80ml) apricot kernel or sunflower oil

Additive:

- 6 drops grapefruit seed extract (GSE), optional

Essential Oil:

- 10–12 drops jasmine absolute

HOW TO MAKE

1. Crush your jasmine petals with a mortar and pestle, in a coffee grinder, or with your hands to create a coarse powder.
2. Mix the exfoliants until they are distributed evenly.
3. Melt the coconut oil for 15 seconds in the microwave and add it to the exfoliants. Then add the apricot kernel oil, GSE (if using), and essential oils.
4. Stir until fully incorporated. It should have the consistency of glistening wet sand.
5. Spoon into the jars and cap them.

HOW TO USE

In the shower after cleansing, massage the scrub all over your skin. Once you rinse, your skin will be soft and hydrated, with no need for lotion. You can also use this scrub in the bath for deeply relaxing and restorative skin rejuvenation.

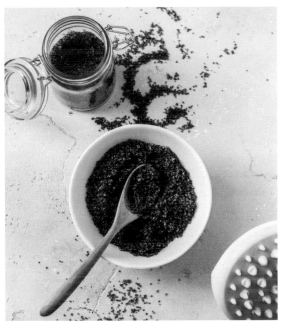

Simply crush the jasmine petals in your hand to make a powder for this scrub.

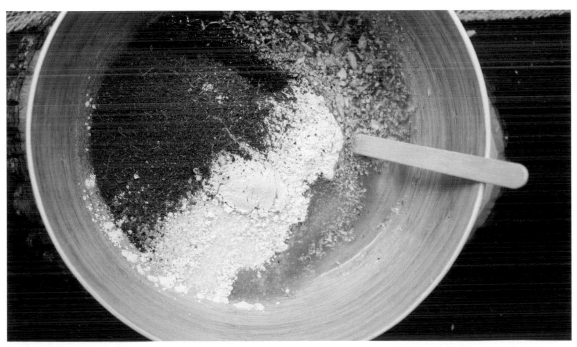

Making body scrubs is as simple as combining your ingredients in a bowl and stirring them to combine.

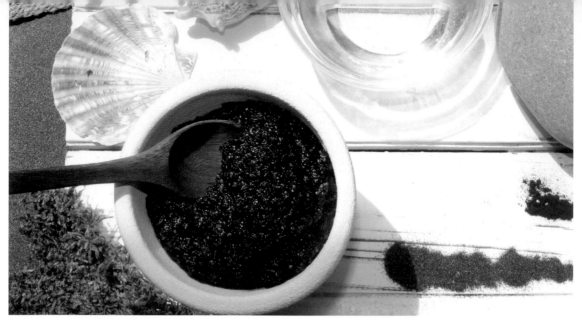

This scrub captures the essence of the ocean with a combination of salt, sand, and seaweed.

OCEANA SANDS SCRUB

MAKES 8 OUNCES (250ML)

Growing up in California but now living in New Mexico, sometimes my body viscerally craves the ocean. This vibrant and invigorating scrub is like a morning dip in the waves with sand, salt, seaweed, and the bright essential oils of eucalyptus and peppermint. The minerals and nutrients in this mix help fortify your skin as the scrub gently exfoliates and moisturizes, waking up both body and mind.

EQUIPMENT

- Mixing bowl
- Wooden stir stick or stirring spoon
- Glass jars

INGREDIENTS

Exfoliant Base:

- 1 cup (250ml) fine sea salt
- 2 tablespoons (30ml) sand (I used black sand, but you can use any color or type you prefer)
- 1 teaspoon (5ml) powdered kelp or spirulina

Dispersants:

- ½ cup (125ml) sunflower oil
- 2 tablespoons (30ml) mango butter

Essential Oils:

- ⅛ teaspoon (0.5ml) eucalyptus
- ⅛ teaspoon (0.5ml) peppermint

HOW TO MAKE

1. Mix the exfoliants until distributed evenly.
2. Melt the mango butter for 15 seconds in the microwave and add to the exfoliants. Then add the sunflower oil and essential oils.
3. Stir until fully incorporated. It should have the consistency of glistening wet sand. Spoon into the jars and cap them.

HOW TO USE

In the shower after cleansing, massage the scrub all over your skin in circles. Rinse off with a loofah or washcloth.

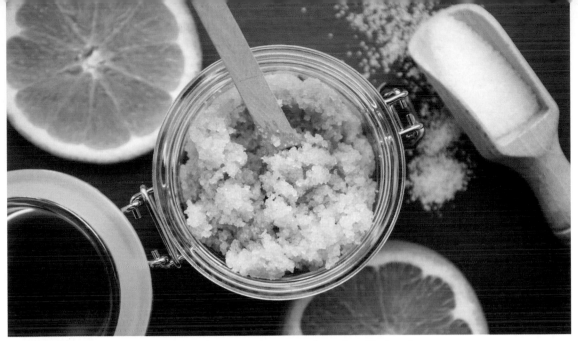

Use this fresh and fruity sugar scrub after cleansing to leave your skin soft and hydrated.

TANGERINE SUGAR SCRUB
MAKES 8 OUNCES (250ML)

This sweet treat leaves your skin glistening and hydrated and has exfoliating and softening effects when used after cleansing in the shower. Sugar contains minerals that enrich, promoting healthy, soft, and smooth skin.

EQUIPMENT
- Mixing bowl
- Wooden stir stick or stirring spoon
- Glass jars

INGREDIENTS
Exfoliants:
- 1 cup (250ml) organic white sugar
- 1 tablespoon (15ml) pink clay

Dispersants:
- ⅓ cup (80ml) sunflower oil
- 1 tablespoon (15ml) coconut oil
- 1 teaspoon (5ml) aloe vera gel
- 1 teaspoon (5ml) glycerin

Essential Oil:
- 2 teaspoons (10ml) tangerine

HOW TO MAKE
1. Mix the exfoliants until they are evenly distributed.
2. Melt the coconut oil for 15 seconds in the microwave and add it to the exfoliants. Then add the sunflower oil, aloe vera, glycerin, and essential oil. Stir until fully incorporated. The scrub should have the consistency of glistening wet sand.
3. Spoon into the jars and cap them.

HOW TO USE
In the shower after cleansing, massage the scrub all over your skin in circles. Once you rinse, your skin will be left soft and hydrated, without any need for lotion. If your scrub dries out over time, simply add a bit more sunflower oil to rehydrate it.

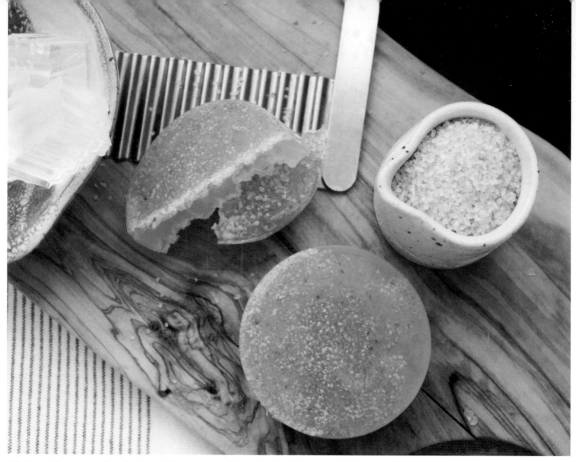

Adding salt to your glycerin bars brings a natural touch of exfoliation to slough off dead skin and reveal newer, fresher skin.

SALTED PINK GRAPEFRUIT BAR
MAKES TWO 4-OUNCE (113G) BARS

This little pink-tinged bar matches the gentle exfoliation of sea salt with the cleansing power of olive oil glycerin soap. With the light and heavenly smell of pink grapefruit, this may become your go-to bar for daily cleansing that has just a little something extra.

EQUIPMENT
- Two 4-ounce (113g) soap molds
- Kitchen scale
- Glass measuring cup
- Stirring spoon

INGREDIENTS
Base:
- 8-ounce (225g) clear olive oil glycerin soap block
- ½ cup (125ml) white or pink sea salt

Essential Oil:
- 1 tablespoon (15ml) pink grapefruit

HOW TO MAKE

1. Weigh the glycerin and then cut it into ½" (12.7mm) cubes and place it in the measuring cup. Microwave the cubes until melted, stopping to stir every 1 minute.
2. Add the essential oil and stir to incorporate.
3. Pour into soap molds, leaving about ⅛" (3mm) space at the top.
4. Scoop ¼ cup (60ml) of pink salt into each bar mold (it will sink to the bottom). Once the bars cool a bit and have a tacky surface, you can also sprinkle more salt on top if you want.
5. Let sit for 2 to 4 hours or overnight.
6. Place in the freezer for 20 minutes and then pop out onto a plate, a cutting board, or wax paper.

HOW TO USE

Use in the shower to cleanse and gently exfoliate, or as a hand cleansing bar at the sink.

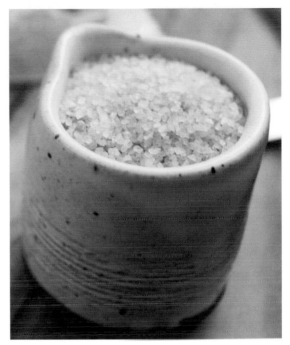

I like using pink salt, but feel free to experiment with different colors from around the world.

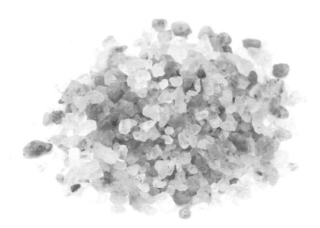

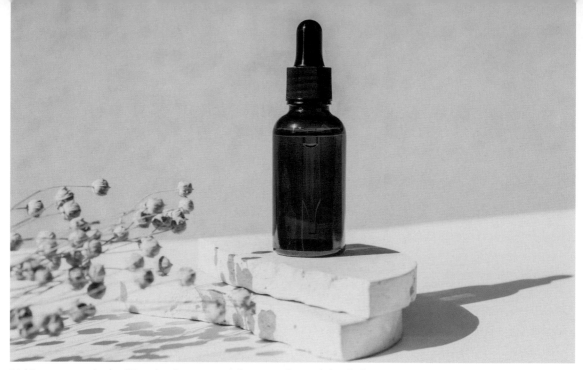

Making your own body oil is a simple process of choosing a base oil that feels good on your skin, and then adding your chosen essential oils for their aromatic and health benefits.

POMEGRANATE BODY OIL
MAKES 8 OUNCES (250ML)

Leave your skin glistening and happy with this allover body oil you can use after showering or for massages. Pomegranate seed oil is anti-inflammatory, antimicrobial, restorative, and hydrating without being overly oily. Geranium essential oil is brightening and full of antioxidants that fight free radicals and skin damage.

EQUIPMENT
- 8-ounce (250ml) glass bottle
- Funnel
- Ingredients

Base:
- 4 ounces (125ml) pomegranate seed oil
- 4 ounces (125ml) sunflower or olive oil

Essential Oil:
- 1½ teaspoons (7ml) geranium

HOW TO MAKE
1. Pour the base oils into the glass bottle, then add the essential oil.
2. Cap and shake the bottle to blend.

HOW TO USE
Massage into your skin after a shower or use to massage your feet, hands, arms, or anywhere that needs some extra TLC. The bright aroma of geranium and the rich texture of pomegranate seed oil give soothing, long-lasting massage results.

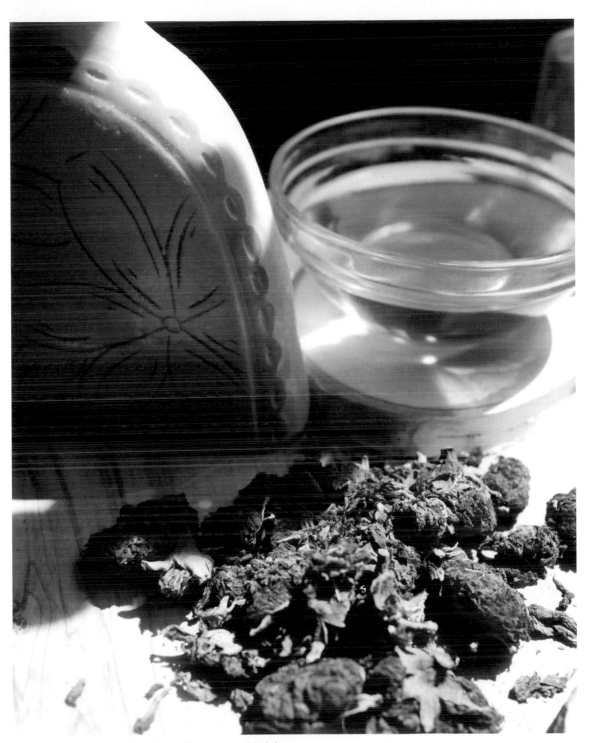

Pomegranates create a rich oil that is luxurious and indulgent.

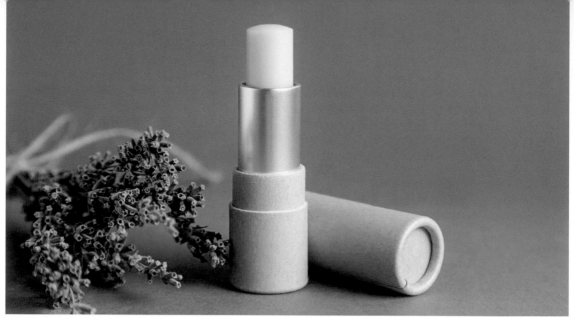

This lotion stick provides on-the-go hydration and relaxation.

LAVENDER LOTION STICK

MAKES FOUR 2.37-OUNCE (70ML) TUBES

Lavender might be the single most popular essential oil because of its ability to induce relaxation as well as soothe anxiety, depression, and insomnia, and heal skin with its anti-inflammatory esters. This lotion stick delivers hydration, healing, and mood boosting all in one small, transportable package you can take along to the gym, work, or pretty much anywhere, keeping you grounded *and* hydrated wherever life takes you.

EQUIPMENT

- Glass measuring cup
- Four 2.37-ounce (70ml) paper push-up tubes
- Wooden stir stick

INGREDIENTS

Base:

- ½ cup (125ml) mango butter or lavender-infused soy butter
- ½ cup (60g) candelilla wax
- ¼ cup (60ml) avocado oil
- 2 tablespoons (30ml) coconut oil

Essential Oil:

- 1 teaspoon (5ml) lavender

HOW TO MAKE

1. Add the base ingredients to the measuring cup and microwave 30 seconds at a time, stirring in between, until the wax and butter are melted.
2. Add the essential oil and stir to incorporate it.
3. Pour slowly into the tubes until they are full. They should have a subtle rounding at the top.
4. Let sit for 1 to 2 hours before capping.

HOW TO USE

This convenient lotion stick makes it easy to carry healing and hydration with you wherever you go. Keep it in your purse to hydrate your hands and face, under your eyes, your feet, or anywhere you need skin softening, smoothing, and the aromatherapeutic benefit of pure lavender essential oil. It serves to soothe mild skin irritations as well.

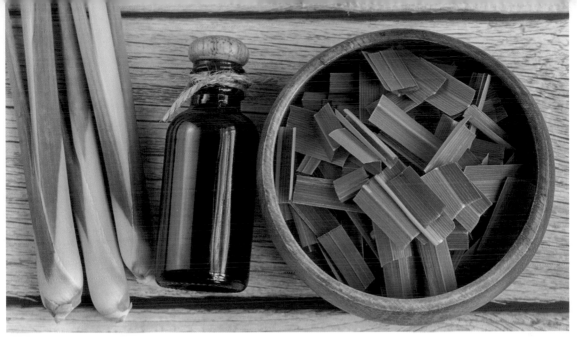

Lemongrass essential oil has antianxiety and antidepressant qualities to lift your mood and get your day off to a good start.

LEMONGRASS BODY WASH
MAKES 8 OUNCES (250ML)

The refreshing and soothing scent of lemongrass above a hint of lavender makes for a delightful way to start your day. Healthful ingredients that offer softening and vitamins infuse the castile soap, while the lemongrass essential oil adds vibrancy and mood-balancing effects. The oils add hydration, which makes this perfectly suited to use as hair shampoo, too!

EQUIPMENT
- 8-ounce (250ml) bottle
- Funnel

INGREDIENTS
Base:
- 8 ounces (250ml) lavender-infused castile soap
- 1 tablespoon (15ml) fractionated coconut oil
- 1 tablespoon (15ml) glycerin
- 2 teaspoons (10ml) olive or avocado oil
- 1 teaspoon (5ml) vitamin E oil

Essential Oil:
- 1 teaspoon (5ml) lemongrass

HOW TO MAKE
1. Pour the castile soap into the bottle and add the essential oil.
2. Cap and shake the bottle to blend.

HOW TO USE
Shake before each use. Pour 1–2 teaspoons (5–10ml) onto a loofah or washcloth or into the palm of your hands and wash wherever desired.

TIP: If you only have unscented castile soap available, you can still make this lovely body wash—simply add ½ teaspoon (2.5ml) lavender essential oil.

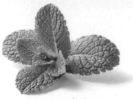

PEPPERMINT FOOT RUB
MAKES 8 OUNCES (250ML)

This treat for your tootsies is infused with arnica oil, sea salt, and both the tea and essential oil of peppermint to create a pain-reducing, restorative treatment. Thick and rich, it allows for a long and deep massage to reinvigorate tired feet. A daily self massage will help keep your feet limber and prevent pain. *See Emulsion Tips on page 67.*

EQUIPMENT
- Small glass bowl
- Glass measuring cup
- Thermometer, optional
- Smoothie blender
- Measuring spoons
- Wooden stir stick
- Glass jars
- Double boiler, optional

INGREDIENTS
Water Phase:
- ¼ cup (60ml) aloe vera
- ¼ cup (60ml) peppermint tea
- ⅛ teaspoon (0.5ml) citric acid
- 1½ teaspoons (7ml) glycerin

Oil Phase:
- 2 tablespoons (30ml) mango butter
- 1 tablespoon (15ml) coconut oil
- 3 tablespoons (21g) e-wax
- 1 tablespoon (15ml) arnica oil
- 1 teaspoon (5ml) jojoba
- ⅛ teaspoon (0.5 ml) stearic acid

Additive:
- ¼ cup (60ml) fine sea salt

Essential Oil:
- 2 teaspoons (10ml) peppermint

Preservative:
- ½ teaspoon (2.5ml) Germaben II

HOW TO MAKE

Prepare the Water Phase
1. Combine water phase ingredients in a glass bowl and heat in the microwave for 1 minute until the citric acid is dissolved.
2. Stir and test the temperature with your thermometer. If it's not yet at 160°F–170°F (71°–77°C), microwave for 1 more minute and then set it aside.

Prepare the Oil Phase
1. Melt all the oil phase ingredients in a double boiler (or in the microwave, 1 minute at a time, stirring in between). Stir until all the butters are melted.
2. Heat to the same temperature as the water phase, letting cool if needed to reach the correct temperature range.

Blend the Phases
1. When phases are within the correct temperature range and are approximately the same temperature, pour the water phase into the small blender.
2. Add the oil phase—it should immediately turn white.
3. Blend for 5 to 10 seconds until fully combined.
4. Open the blender and allow the mixture to cool to 140°F (60°C). A temperature above that can compromise the preservative.
5. Add the essential oil, salt, and preservative, and blend for 5 to 10 seconds more.
6. Pour or spoon the mixture into glass jars and allow it to cool and thicken before capping them.

HOW TO USE
Massage a liberal amount into your feet slowly, giving special attention to your arches, the tops of your feet, and between your toes.

TIP: If you don't have peppermint tea, you can swap in peppermint hydrosol or distilled water instead.

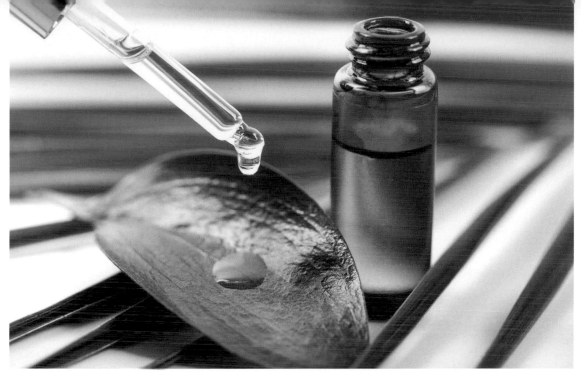

This luxurious oil leaves hair silky, sleek, and protected.

BERGAMOT SMOOTHING HAIR OIL
MAKES 1 OUNCE (30ML)

To smooth and tame thick or unruly hair, easily make your own smoothing oil. With the refreshing aroma of bergamot essential oil, this hair oil also leaves your hair smelling clean and fresh.

EQUIPMENT
- 1-ounce (30ml) glass dropper bottle
- Measuring spoons
- Funnel

INGREDIENTS
Base:
- 1 tablespoon (15ml) olive oil
- 1 teaspoon (5ml) argan oil
- 1 teaspoon (5ml) jojoba
- 1 teaspoon (5ml) pomegranate seed oil
- ⅛ teaspoon (0.5ml) glycerin
- 6 drops vitamin E oil

Essential Oil:
- ¼ teaspoon (1.25ml) bergamot

HOW TO MAKE
1. Pour all the ingredients into the bottle using the funnel.
2. Cap the bottle and swirl gently to incorporate.

HOW TO USE
Shake 3 to 5 drops into the palms of your hands and distribute onto the ends of clean, dry hair. Comb through and style as desired.

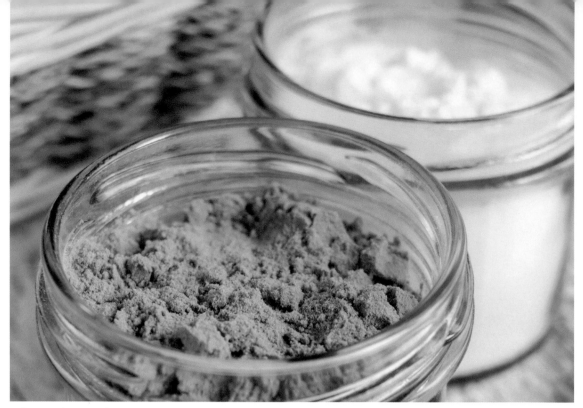

Color-matched dry shampoo is perfect for days when you need to get ready quickly or for a post-gym refresh.

CLARY SAGE DRY SHAMPOO
MAKES 4 OUNCES (125ML)

It's easy to make your own oil-absorbing powder to keep your hair fresh and clean in between shampoos. The base recipe is for light to medium hair colors, but I've listed additional ingredients on page 125 so you can customize it for red and brunette tones.

EQUIPMENT
- Mixing bowl
- Stirring spoon
- Measuring spoons
- Measuring cup
- Shaker tube or can

INGREDIENTS
Base:
- ½ cup (125ml) arrowroot powder or corn starch
- 2 tablespoons (30ml) raw cacao powder
- 2 tablespoons (30ml) bentonite or kaolin clay
- 1 tablespoon (15ml) rose petal powder
- 1 tablespoon (15ml) baking soda

Essential Oil:
- ¼ teaspoon (1.25ml) clary sage or geranium

COLOR MATCHING

To better match your own hair color, use these additives in small quantities, building color ¼ teaspoon (1.25ml) at a time to deepen the hue of your dry shampoo.

- Dark brown/black: activated charcoal
- Red/light brown: cinnamon powder

DRY SHAMPOO SCENT ALTERNATIVES

You can always make this recipe your own by using ¼ teaspoon (1.25ml) of your favorite scent (try using the one that makes you happiest).

HOW TO MAKE

1. Measure all the ingredients into your mixing bowl. Stir to incorporate, pressing out any clumps with the back of your spoon.
2. Spoon the mixture into your shaker can and cap with the lid.

HOW TO USE

Sprinkle onto your scalp near the roots or dab on with a makeup brush. Use your fingers or a comb to incorporate (see photos below).

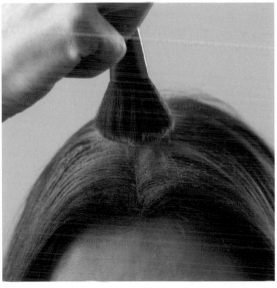

Use a makeup brush to dab dry shampoo near your roots.

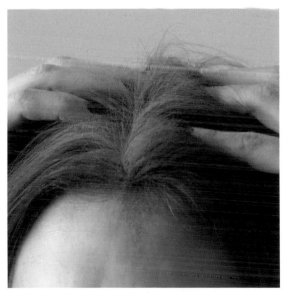

Evenly distribute the powder with your fingers.

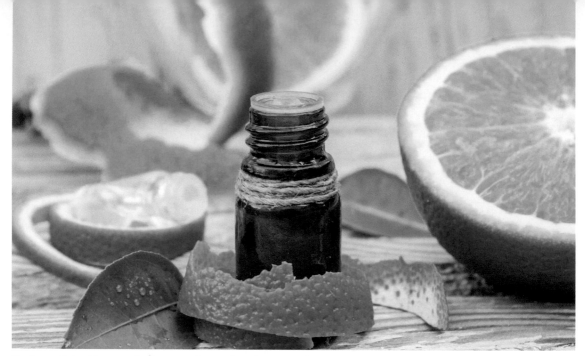

The base oils in this cream hydrate your hair to form bouncy curls. The sweet orange essential oil and vanilla absolute create a soft, sensual scent.

SWEET ORANGE CURL CREAM
MAKES 8 OUNCES (113G)

Just say no to crunch! This cream creates soft curls without the crispness often found in other curl creams. *See Emulsion Tips on page 67.*

EQUIPMENT
- Small glass bowl
- Glass measuring cup
- Thermometer, optional
- 8-ounce (113g) pump bottle, jar, or tin
- Kitchen scale
- Measuring spoons
- Wooden stir stick
- Double boiler, optional

TIP: To simplify this recipe, use just one type of oil (just olive, coconut, or camellia) and omit the orange wax.

INGREDIENTS
Water Phase:
- 8 ounces (250ml) distilled water
- 1 tablespoon (15ml) aloe vera gel
- 1 tablespoon (15ml) glycerin
- 1 teaspoon (5ml) citric acid

Oil Phase:
- 1 tablespoon (15ml) camellia tea seed oil
- 1 tablespoon (15ml) olive oil
- 1 tablespoon (15ml) coconut oil
- 1 tablespoon (15ml) mango butter
- 2 tablespoons (14g) e-wax
- 1 tablespoon (15ml) orange wax
- 1 teaspoon (5ml) stearic acid
- 5 drops vitamin E oil

Essential Oils:
- ¼ teaspoon (1.25ml) vanilla absolute
- ½ teaspoon (2.5ml) sweet orange

Preservative:
- ½ teaspoon (2.5ml) Germaben II

HOW TO MAKE

Prepare the Water Phase

1. Combine water phase ingredients in a glass bowl and heat in the microwave for 1 minute until the citric acid is dissolved.
2. Stir and test the temperature with your thermometer. If it's not yet at 160°F–170°F (71°–77°C), microwave for 1 more minute and then set it aside.

Prepare the Oil Phase

1. Melt all the oil phase ingredients in a double boiler (or in the microwave, 1 minute at a time, stirring in between). Stir until all the butters are melted.
2. Heat to the same temperature as the water phase, letting cool if needed to reach the correct temperature range.

Blend the Phases

1. When phases are within the correct temperature range and are approximately the same temperature, pour the water phase into the small blender.
2. Add the oil phase—it should immediately turn white.
3. Blend for 5 to 10 seconds until fully combined.
4. Open the blender and allow the mixture to cool to 140°F (60°C). A temperature above that can compromise the preservative.
5. Add the essential oil and preservative, and blend for 5 to 10 seconds more.
6. Pour or spoon the mixture into tins or glass jars. Allow it to cool and thicken before capping them.

HOW TO USE

Depending on your hair thickness and length, apply 1 teaspoon (5ml) to 1 tablespoon (15ml) of cream to the underside and ends of wet or damp hair. Comb it through and then twist or scrunch as desired before letting your hair air dry.

TIP: Even though this is a curl cream, I also use it when I blow-dry my hair straight—I love the way it makes my hair soft and smooth!

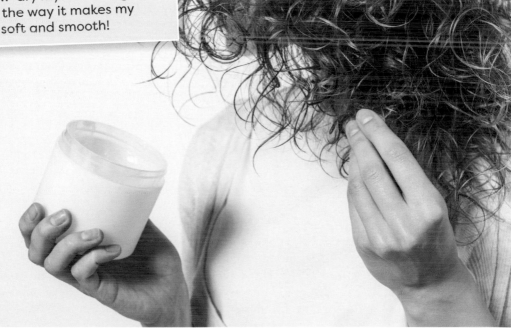

This light cream thoroughly hydrates curls to create soft, natural texture.

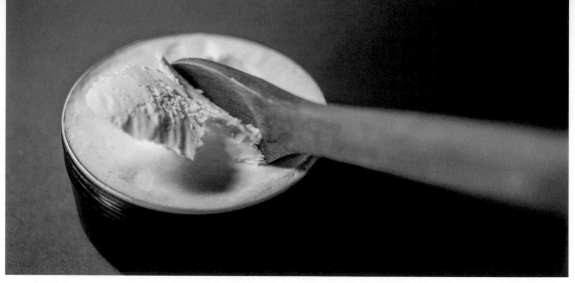

Cocoa butter leaves your hair soft and smooth, while giving you control over your style.

COCOA HAIR STYLING BUTTER

MAKES 4 OUNCES (125ML)

A little of this butter goes a long way! Use it to style, scrunch, spike, or whatever else your heart desires. This butter also protects your hair during heat styling.

EQUIPMENT

- Glass measuring cup
- 4-ounce (113g) tin or jar
- Kitchen scale
- Measuring spoons
- Wooden stir stick

INGREDIENTS

Base:

- ½ cup (60g) cocoa butter
- 1 tablespoon (15ml) coconut oil
- 1 tablespoon (15ml) argan oil
- 1 teaspoon (5ml) jojoba
- 6 drops vitamin E oil, optional
- 1 tablespoon (15ml) aloe vera gel

Essential Oils:

- 16 drops orange
- 6 drops rosemary

HOW TO MAKE

1. Weigh the cocoa butter and place it in a measuring cup.
2. Add the base oils and jojoba to a measuring cup, and microwave for 1 minute. Stop to stir. If needed, microwave for a few more seconds—stop while there are still small, unmelted pieces so as not to overheat, and then stir until fully melted.
3. Add the aloe vera gel and essential oils and stir to incorporate.
4. Pour into your tin or jar and let sit for 2 to 4 hours until solidified. (If the weather is hot, put the styling butter in the fridge to solidify.) Cap.

HOW TO USE

Smear a very small amount on your finger and rub it in the palm of your hands until the butter melts. Apply it to the underside and ends of wet or dry hair, and then comb or style as desired. Start with less—you can always add more, and a little goes a long way. Also use before heat styling to protect your hair.

FRANKINCENSE SHAVING CREAM
MAKES 8 OUNCES (250ML)

Treat yourself to a luxurious shave with this whipped cream that soothes and protects even the most delicate skin. The essential oil provides nourishment and healing properties. Double the quantity to make plenty for yourself and for gifting to friends. *See Emulsion Tips on page 67.*

EQUIPMENT
- Small glass bowl
- Glass measuring cup
- Thermometer, optional
- Kitchen scale
- Smoothie blender
- Glass jars or tins
- Double boiler, optional

INGREDIENTS

Water Phase:
- ¼ cup (60ml) lavender hydrosol or distilled water
- ¼ cup (60ml) aloe vera gel
- 1½ teaspoons (8ml) glycerin
- ⅛ teaspoon (0.5ml) citric acid

Oil Phase:
- 2 tablespoons (30ml) mango butter
- 2 tablespoons (30ml) jojoba
- 3 tablespoons (21g) e-wax
- 1 tablespoon (15ml) coconut oil
- ⅛ teaspoon (0.5 ml) stearic acid

Essential Oil:
- 1 teaspoon (5ml) frankincense, cedarwood, or sandalwood

Preservative:
- ½ teaspoon (2.5ml) Germaben II

HOW TO MAKE

Prepare the Water Phase
1. Combine water phase ingredients in a glass bowl and heat in the microwave for 1 minute until the citric acid is dissolved.
2. Stir and test the temperature with your thermometer. If it's not yet at 160°F–170°F (71°–77°C), microwave for 1 more minute and then set it aside.

Prepare the Oil Phase
1. Melt all the oil phase ingredients in a double boiler (or in the microwave, 1 minute at a time, stirring in between). Stir until all the butters are melted.
2. Heat to the same temperature as the water phase, letting cool if needed to reach the correct temperature range.

Blend the Phases
1. When phases are within the correct temperature range and are approximately the same temperature, pour the water phase into the small blender.
2. Add the oil phase—it should immediately turn white.
3. Blend for 5 to 10 seconds until fully combined.
4. Open the blender and allow the mixture to cool to 140°F (60°C). A temperature above that can compromise the preservative.
5. Add the essential oil and preservative, and blend for 5 to 10 seconds more.
6. Pour or spoon the mixture into tins or glass jars and allow it to cool and thicken before capping them.

HOW TO USE
Spread over your skin before shaving. Shave and then rinse or wipe off with a warm, wet towel.

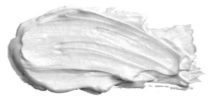

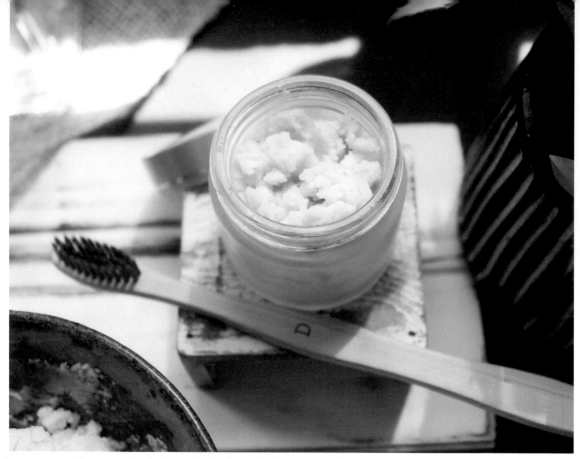

Leave toxins and preservatives behind with this naturally cleansing tooth polish made from just a few healthful ingredients.

PEPPERMINT TOOTH POLISH

MAKES 8 OUNCES (250ML)

Reach a new level of clean for your teeth and your whole mouth with this super-polishing, naturally bacteria-battling, minty fresh tooth polish. Make one large jar or fill smaller jars to gift to your loved ones.

EQUIPMENT
- Mixing bowl
- Stirring spoon
- Glass jars

INGREDIENTS

Dry:
- 1 cup (250ml) baking soda
- ¼ cup (60ml) fine calcium carbonate powder
- 2 tablespoons (30ml) white clay

Wet:
- ¼ cup (60ml) fractionated coconut oil
- 2 tablespoons (30ml) glycerin
- 1½ teaspoons (7ml) food-grade hydrogen peroxide

Essential Oil:
- ¾ teaspoon (3.5ml) peppermint

HOW TO MAKE

1. Mix the dry ingredients until fully incorporated.
2. Mix the wet ingredients until fully incorporated.
3. Combine the wet and dry ingredients.
4. Add the essential oil and stir with a spoon, pressing out each lump until the mixture is smooth and uniform. If it feels too dry, add a touch more melted coconut oil and blend until you are happy with the consistency.
5. Spoon into glass jars, pressing the paste firmly to the bottom as you fill.

HOW TO USE

Add a pea-sized amount to your toothbrush and brush your teeth as normal. Rinse. Enjoy polished teeth and fresh breath, naturally!

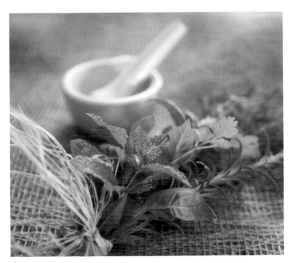

Peppermint essential oil is the perfect ingredient for creating an all-day fresh feeling.

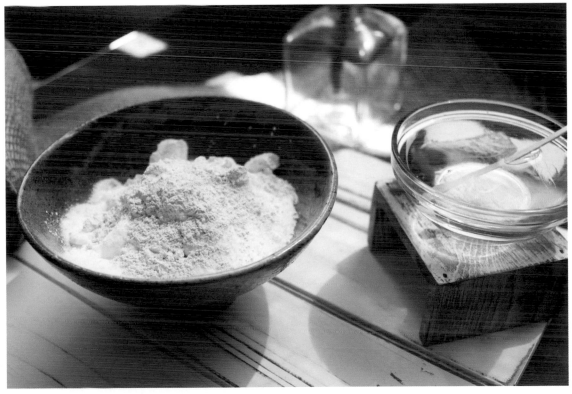

This tooth polish naturally leaves your teeth squeaky clean and your breath fresh.

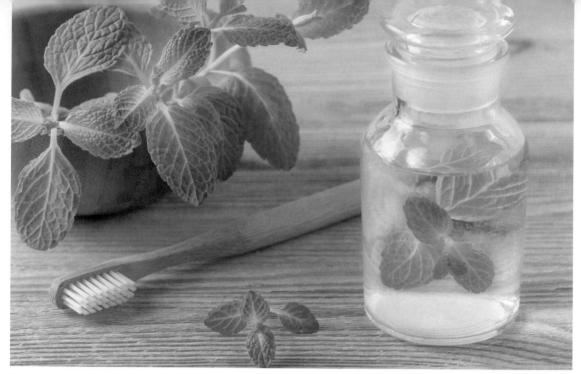

This natural mouthwash cleanses and soothes your gums as it freshens your breath.

MENTHOLATED MOUTH RINSE
MAKES 8 OUNCES (250ML)

This refreshing mouthwash won't burn like commercial brands, instead giving a gentle and refreshing lift, leaving your mouth clean and fresh from the eucalyptus water and menthol essential oil. The coconut oil is a natural antibacterial agent and offers a nice skin-soothing texture.

EQUIPMENT

- 8-ounce (250ml) glass bottle
- Measuring spoons
- Funnel

INGREDIENTS

Base:

- 1 cup (250ml) eucalyptus hydrosol, peppermint hydrosol, or distilled water
- 1 teaspoon (5ml) fractionated coconut oil

Essential Oil:

- ¼–½ teaspoon (1.25–2.5ml) menthol or peppermint (start with the lesser amount if using menthol as it's very strong)

HOW TO MAKE

1. Add all the ingredients to the bottle and close the cap.
2. Shake to incorporate.

HOW TO USE

After brushing or anytime you need a refreshing feeling, swish approximately 1 tablespoon (15ml) in your mouth for a few seconds and spit it out. Shake well before each use.

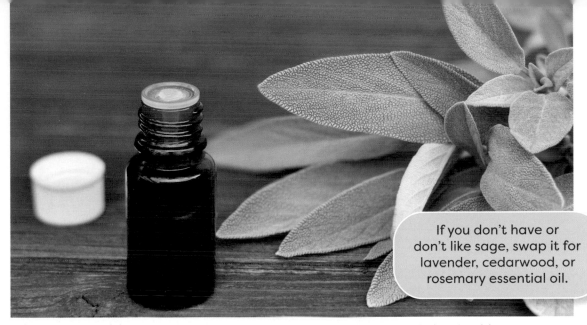

If you don't have or don't like sage, swap it for lavender, cedarwood, or rosemary essential oil.

Sage (*Salvia lavandifolia*) essential oil is antiseptic, calming, and mood-lifting, adding to the benefits of this grooming balm.

SAGE EYEBROW TAMING BALM
MAKES 1 OUNCE (30ML)

This little balm has the skin-soothing properties of sage, an evergreen in the mint family that's native to the Mediterranean and prolific in the southwest United States. Enhanced with natural hydrators like coconut oil, cocoa butter, and aloe vera, this little tin will keep your eyebrows where you want them.

EQUIPMENT
- Glass measuring cup
- Measuring spoons
- 1-ounce (30ml) tin or glass jar

INGREDIENTS
Base:
- 1 tablespoon (5g) candelilla wax
- 1 tablespoon (5g) unrefined cocoa butter
- 1 tablespoon (15ml) virgin coconut oil
- 1 teaspoon (5ml) aloe vera gel
- 1 teaspoon (5ml) glycerin

Essential Oil:
- ⅛ teaspoon (0.5ml) sage

HOW TO MAKE
1. Melt the cocoa butter in the microwave, stirring after 1 minute, then heating for an additional 30 seconds. When it's almost fully melted, stir until all the pieces are dissolved.
2. Add the coconut oil and stir to melt.
3. Add the other ingredients and stir to incorporate.
4. Pour into the glass jar and allow to sit for 1 hour before capping.
5. Allow it to sit for at least 2 hours or overnight to solidify before first use.

HOW TO USE
Smooth a bit over your eyebrows after combing to keep them tamed.

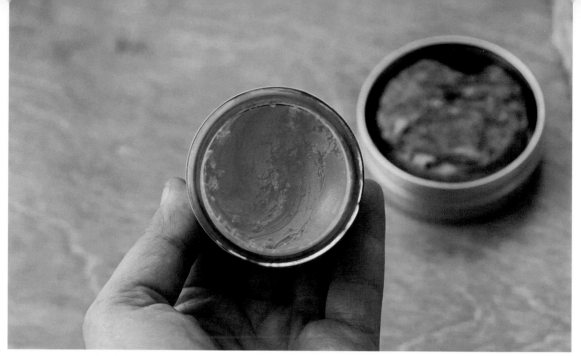

Many commercial deodorants are harsh on delicate skin. This deodorant soothes your skin as it fights bacteria and odor.

CHARCOAL ANTIBACTERIAL DEODORANT
MAKES THREE 2.37-OUNCE (70ML) PAPER TUBES

Organic and effective, this deodorant features activated charcoal—a magic ingredient that absorbs dirt, toxins, heavy metals, and chemicals to keep them off your skin—plus a host of other natural antibacterial ingredients, including orange peel powder, arrowroot powder, kaolin clay, and the antibacterial essential oils of rosemary, orange, lemon, and clove.

EQUIPMENT
- Mixing bowl
- Wooden stir stick or stirring spoon
- Glass measuring cup
- Measuring spoons
- Paper tubes or glass jars

INGREDIENTS
Wet:
- ⅓ cup (80ml) hemp butter, mango butter, or shea butter
- ¼ cup (60ml) coconut oil
- ½ cup (60g) candelilla wax
- 3 tablespoons (45ml) sunflower seed oil
- ⅛ teaspoon (0.5ml) vitamin E oil
- 12 drops grapefruit seed extract (GSE), optional

Dry:
- 1 teaspoon (5ml) white kaolin clay
- 1 teaspoon (5ml) arrowroot
- 1 teaspoon (5ml) baking soda
- 1 teaspoon (5ml) activated charcoal
- ½ teaspoon (2.5ml) orange peel powder

Essential Oils:
- ⅛ teaspoon (0.5 ml) rosemary
- 1 teaspoon (5ml) orange
- ½ teaspoon (2.5ml) lemon
- 6 drops clove

HOW TO MAKE

1. Combine the wet ingredients and melt in the microwave for 1 minute. Stop to stir. If needed, microwave again, stopping every 30 seconds to stir until just before the mixture is liquefied (stop before fully liquefied to avoid overheating).
2. Add the dry ingredients and stir for about 30 seconds until the dry ingredients are dissolved and fully combined.
3. Add the essential oils and stir thoroughly.
4. While the mixture is still hot, give it one last stir from the bottom to incorporate any charcoal and other dry ingredients that might have fallen to the bottom.
5. Pour into tubes or jars and let set 1 to 2 hours before capping. To ensure they are completely solid, let sit overnight before first use.

HOW TO USE

Use under your arms or wherever you prefer after showering to stay fresh. Reapply as needed.

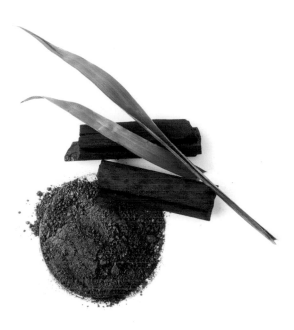

Activated charcoal binds to odor-causing bacteria, helping to eliminate it.

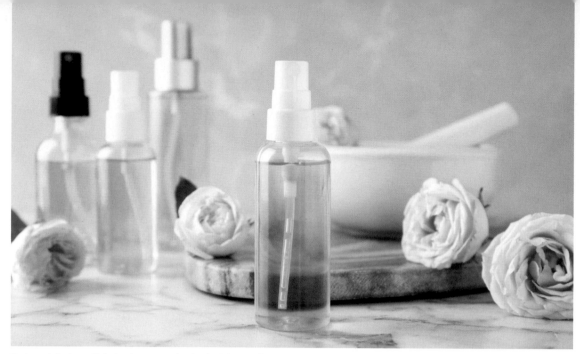

Hydrosols help to lightly cleanse and refresh delicate skin, and there are many lovely options to choose from.

PERSONAL TOILETRY MIST

MAKES 1-OUNCE (30ML) SPRAY

For a fresher and more thorough clean after attending to the call of nature, keep this mist in your purse or in your lavatory. I used rose hydrosol, but you can use any floral water—chamomile, lavender, or calendula also make great choices. The aloe, calendula, and glycerin offer softening and soothing properties, while the floral water cleans naturally and has gentle antibacterial properties.

EQUIPMENT

- 1-ounce (30ml) spray bottle
- Small funnel
- Measuring spoons

INGREDIENTS

- 1 tablespoon (15ml) rose hydrosol or other floral water of choice
- 2 teaspoons (10ml) witch hazel
- ½ teaspoon (2.5ml) aloe vera
- ¼ teaspoon (1.25ml) glycerin
- ¼ teaspoon (1.25ml) calendula oil
- Scant ⅛ teaspoon (0.5ml) citric acid, optional preservative

HOW TO MAKE

1. Add each ingredient to the bottle using a funnel.
2. Close and tighten the top, then swirl to incorporate.

HOW TO USE

Spray onto toilet paper and wipe as normal. Alternatively, this recipe is gentle enough to spray directly on the skin after wiping.

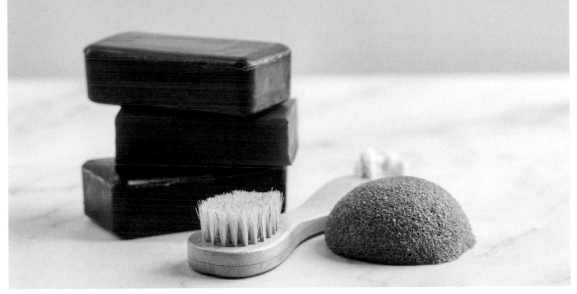

This bar easily scrubs away dirt and grease while soothing and protecting your skin.

DE-GRIMING LEMON HAND SOAP BAR

MAKES TWO 4-OUNCE (113G) BARS

Use this gritty, exfoliating bar to tackle grease and grime on your hands. The extracting and exfoliating powdered pumice, activated charcoal, and clay are countered by the softening and hydrating shea butter glycerin soap to create a well-rounded sink bar to take on the toughest cleansing challenge.

EQUIPMENT

- Two 4-ounce (113g) soap molds
- Kitchen scale
- Glass measuring cup
- Small glass bowl
- Measuring spoon
- Whisk or fork

INGREDIENTS

Base:

- 8-ounce (250ml) shea butter glycerin soap block
- ¼ cup (60ml) fine pumice powder
- 2 tablespoons (30ml) white or green clay
- 1 teaspoon (5ml) activated charcoal

Essential Oil:

- 2 tablespoons (30ml) lemon

HOW TO MAKE

1. Cut glycerin soap into approximately ½" (12.7mm) cubes. Add to a glass measuring cup.
2. Melt the cubes in the microwave, stopping to stir every minute. It usually takes 2–3 minutes to fully melt.
3. While your soap is melting, stir together the clay, pumice, and charcoal.
4. When the soap is almost fully melted, remove it from the microwave, and stir until it's fully melted. (It's always good to stop before it's fully melted so you don't overheat it.)
5. Add in your dry ingredients and the essential oil and whisk to fully incorporate.
6. Pour into the soap molds and let set 4 hours or overnight. To make it easy to remove from the mold, place it in the freezer for 30 minutes before popping it out onto wax paper, a cutting board, or a plate.

HOW TO USE

Keep at your sink to use after gardening or other dirty jobs.

Recyclable tins are the perfect eco-friendly
option for packaging balms and butters.

TOPICAL TREATMENTS AND FIRST AID RECIPES

Life is full of small nicks, cuts, and bruises that are easily treated at home with a few botanical healing and soothing ingredients. Of course, seek medical attention for anything beyond what a home remedy makes sense for, but for those day-to-day irritants, leverage the healing powers of essential oils and keep a few wipes, salves, and balms on hand to apply natural healing without added chemicals.

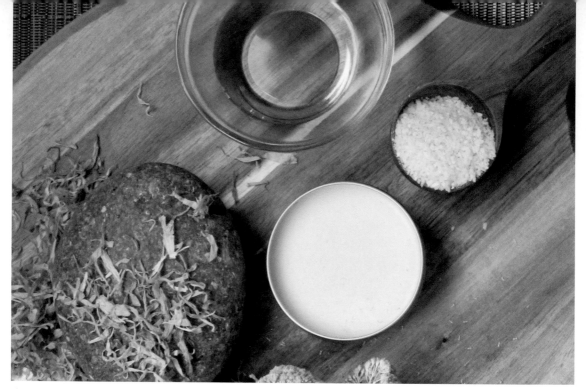

This all-purpose skin salve leverages the healing powers of flowers: calendula, sunflower, helichrysum, and yarrow.

SOOTHING SKIN SALVE

MAKES 4 OUNCES (125ML)

This salve soothes and supports skin health with a plant-based organic balm enhanced with the gentle healing powers of this floral trio of essential oils. The base oils include powerful anti-inflammatory oils like calendula, St. John's wort, arnica, and sea buckthorn, as well as antimicrobial coconut oil, which leaves a protective barrier on the skin.

EQUIPMENT

- Glass measuring cup
- Measuring spoons
- 4-ounce (125ml) tin or multiple smaller tins
- Wooden stir stick

INGREDIENTS

Base:
- ¼ cup (30g) candelilla wax
- ¼ cup (60ml) jojoba
- ¼ cup (60ml) sunflower oil
- ¼ cup (60ml) calendula oil
- 1 tablespoon (15ml) coconut oil
- 1 tablespoon (15ml) hemp butter
- 1 teaspoon (5ml) St. John's wort oil
- 1 teaspoon (5ml) sea buckthorn oil
- 1 teaspoon (5ml) arnica oil

Essential Oils:
- ¼ teaspoon (1.25ml) rose (or use rose in jojoba for a more economical option)
- ¼ teaspoon (1.25ml) helichrysum
- ⅛ teaspoon (0.5ml) blue yarrow

HOW TO MAKE

1. Add all the base ingredients to the measuring cup. Microwave 30 seconds at a time, stirring in between, until almost fully melted, then stir to fully melt the mixture.
2. Add the essential oils and stir again to incorporate.
3. Pour into the tin (or multiple small containers) and let set for 1 to 2 hours before capping and using.

HOW TO USE

Gently apply this multipurpose remedy on dry, cracked, burned, or irritated skin to soothe and heal.

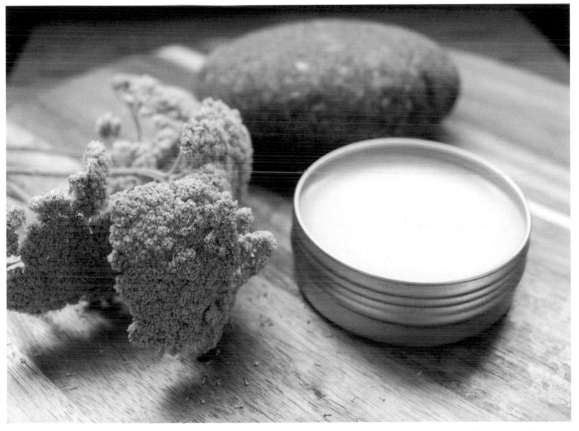

Plant-based candelilla wax, coconut oil, and hemp butter provide additional skin-soothing properties for gentle, effective healing and hydration.

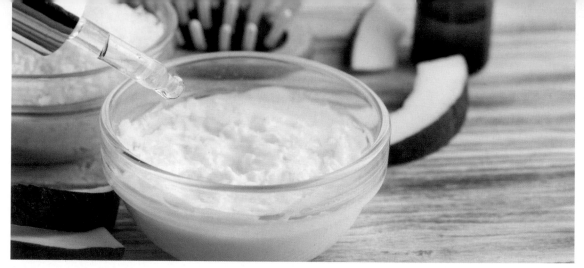

Keeping your skin properly hydrated is the best trick for preserving body art.

TATTOO BUTTER
MAKES APPROXIMATELY 4 OUNCES (113G)

Highlight and help heal tattoos with a naturally rich and healing whipped butter that stays firm but melts easily into the skin. Makes a great gift for the newly inked!

EQUIPMENT
- Glass measuring cup
- Electric mixer
- Mixing spoon
- Mixing bowl (metal or glass)
- Measuring spoons
- 8-ounce (250ml) tin or jar or multiple smaller containers
- Wooden stir stick

INGREDIENTS
Base:
- ¼ cup (60ml) mango butter
- 2 tablespoons (30ml) hemp seed butter
- 2 tablespoons (30ml) lavender-infused soy butter
- 1 tablespoon (15ml) coconut oil
- 1 tablespoon (15ml) calendula oil

Essential Oils:
- 1 teaspoon (5ml) lavender
- ½ teaspoon (2.5ml) frankincense
- ½ teaspoon (2.5ml) tea tree

HOW TO MAKE
1. Add all the base ingredients to the measuring cup. Microwave 30 seconds at a time, stirring in between, until almost fully melted. Then stir to fully melt the mixture.
2. Add the essential oils and stir again to incorporate.
3. Pour into the mixing bowl and place in the freezer for 15 minutes.
4. Take out and scrape the sides (which will be more solid than the center). Whip with the electric mixer for a few seconds until the scraped solids are reincorporated and the cream is a single consistency. Return to the freezer for 10 minutes.
5. Repeat the above step two more times until the mixture reaches a single thick consistency.
6. Scoop into glass or metal containers and cap, label, and enjoy!

HOW TO USE
Rub into your tattoos as desired to help heal fresh tattoos and hydrate and highlight your body art.

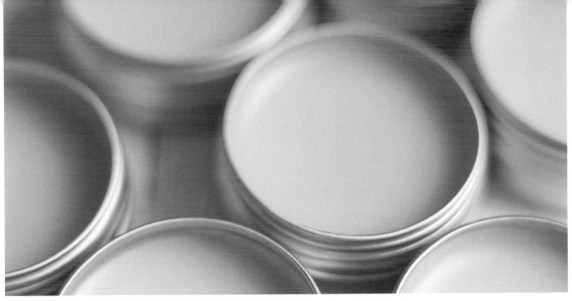

Packaging this balm in tins makes it portable for camping, summer sporting events, picnics, etc.

MOSQUITO REPELLANT BALM
MAKES 8 OUNCES (250ML)

When out in the elements, protect yourself naturally from enemy #1: mosquitos can't stand the aroma of lemon eucalyptus and will leave you in peace. Massage into all exposed skin areas before spending any period of time outdoors during mosquito season.

EQUIPMENT
- Double boiler
- Glass measuring cup
- Measuring spoons
- 8-ounce (250ml) tin or multiple smaller tins
- Wooden stir stick

INGREDIENTS
Base:
- 3 ounces (87ml) hemp butter
- 2 ounces (60ml) shea butter
- 1 tablespoon (5g) candelilla wax
- 1 tablespoon (15ml) sunflower oil

Essential Oils:
- 1 teaspoon (5ml) lemon eucalyptus
- ½ teaspoon (2.5ml) peppermint
- 6 drops vanilla absolute, optional

HOW TO MAKE
1. Add shea butter to the double boiler and melt over medium heat. Once melted, hold at this temperature for 20 minutes to temper (this avoids later crystallization).
2. Add the wax to the measuring cup and microwave for 1 minute. Stir. Repeat as needed in 10-second increments as long as there are still unmelted wax granules. Stir with the stir stick until completely melted.
3. Pour the shea butter into the measuring cup with the wax. Add the essential oil and stir to incorporate.
4. Pour into the tin and let sit for 2 to 4 hours before capping. If it's hot outside, place in the refrigerator to help the mixture set.

HOW TO USE
Spread over any exposed skin before hiking, camping, or enjoying the outdoors in summertime.

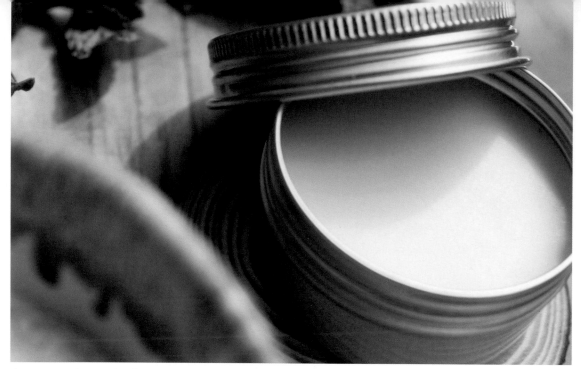
This cream melts into the skin to ease aching muscles.

MENTHOLATED MUSCLE RELIEF CREAM
MAKES 8 OUNCES (250ML)

This organic, light-as-air whipped emulsion is a thick and fluffy mentholated cream to massage into sore or tired muscles, without leaving a thick filmy feeling on the skin. With peppermint hydrosol, aloe vera, mango butter, and menthol essential oil, a little bit of this powerful cream goes a long way. *See Emulsion Tips on page 67.*

EQUIPMENT
- Small glass bowl
- Glass measuring cup
- Thermometer, optional
- Measuring spoons
- 8-ounce (250ml) tin or jar
- Double boiler, optional

INGREDIENTS
Water Phase:
- ¼ cup (60ml) aloe vera gel
- ¼ cup (60ml) peppermint tea, peppermint hydrosol, or distilled water
- 1½ teaspoons (7ml) glycerin
- ⅛ teaspoon (0.5 ml) citric acid
- **Oil Phase:**
- 2 tablespoons (30ml) mango butter

- 1 tablespoon (15ml) coconut oil
- 1 tablespoon (15ml) calendula oil
- 3 tablespoons (21g) e-wax
- ⅛ teaspoon (0.5 ml) stearic acid

Essential Oil:
- 1 teaspoon (5ml) menthol

Preservative:
- ½ teaspoon (2.5ml) Germaben II

HOW TO MAKE

Prepare the Water Phase

1. Combine water phase ingredients in a glass bowl and heat in the microwave for 1 minute until the citric acid is dissolved.
2. Stir and test the temperature with your thermometer. If it's not yet at 160°F–170°F (71°-77°C), microwave for 1 more minute and then set it aside.

Prepare the Oil Phase

1. Melt all the oil phase ingredients in a double boiler (or in the microwave, 1 minute at a time, stirring in between). Stir until all the butters are melted.
2. Heat to the same temperature as the water phase, letting cool if needed to reach the correct temperature range.

Blend the Phases

1. When phases are within the correct temperature range and are approximately the same temperature, pour the water phase into the small blender.
2. Add the oil phase—it should immediately turn white.
3. Blend for 5 to 10 seconds until fully combined.
4. Open the blender and allow the mixture to cool to 140°F (60°C). A temperature above that can compromise the preservative.
5. Add the essential oil and preservative, and blend for 5 to 10 seconds more.
6. Pour or spoon the mixture into tins or glass jars and allow it to cool and thicken before capping them.

HOW TO USE

Massage into sore or tired muscles to soothe, relax, and restore.

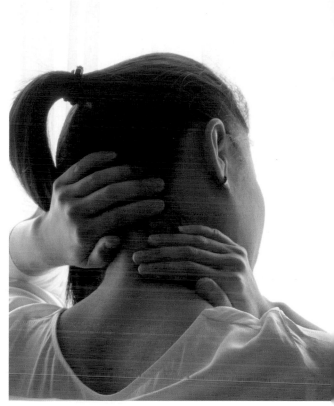

This cream is light enough to be used to soothe everyday aches and pains.

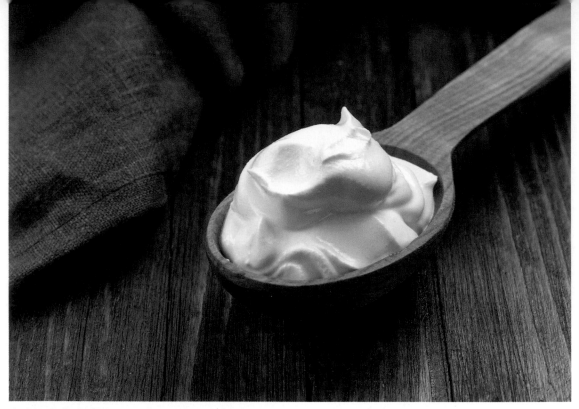

The blend of menthol and deep wood essential oils clears your airways and will help relieve any chest congestion.

DECONGESTANT CHEST RUB

MAKES 8 OUNCES (250ML)

Who needs synthetic, commercial vapor rubs when you can make your own? This leverages the power of menthol essential oil to help soothe and remedy chest congestion naturally. *See Emulsion Tips on page 67.*

EQUIPMENT

- Small glass bowl
- Glass measuring cup
- Thermometer, optional
- Measuring spoons
- 8-ounce (250ml) jar or multiple smaller jars
- Double boiler, optional

INGREDIENTS

Water Phase:
- ¼ cup (60ml) peppermint hydrosol, peppermint tea, or distilled water
- ¼ cup (60ml) aloe vera gel
- 1½ teaspoons (7ml) glycerin
- ½ teaspoon (2.5ml) citric acid

Oil Phase:
- 2 tablespoons (30ml) coconut oil
- 2 tablespoons (30ml) arnica oil
- 1 tablespoon (15ml) mango butter
- 3 tablespoons (21g) e-wax
- ½ teaspoon (2.5ml) stearic acid

Essential Oils:
- 1 teaspoon (5ml) menthol
- ½ teaspoon (2.5ml) black spruce or cypress

Preservative:
- ½ teaspoon (2.5ml) Germaben II

HOW TO MAKE

Prepare the Water Phase

1. Combine water phase ingredients in a glass bowl and heat in the microwave for 1 minute until the citric acid is dissolved.
2. Stir and test the temperature with your thermometer. If it's not yet at 160°F–170°F (71°–77°C), microwave for 1 more minute and then set it aside.

Prepare the Oil Phase

1. Melt all the oil phase ingredients in a double boiler (or in the microwave, 1 minute at a time, stirring in between). Stir until all the butters are melted.
2. Heat to the same temperature as the water phase, letting cool if needed to reach the correct temperature range.

Blend the Phases

1. When phases are within the correct temperature range and are approximately the same temperature, pour the water phase into the small blender.
2. Add the oil phase—it should immediately turn white.
3. Blend for 5 to 10 seconds until fully combined.
4. Open the blender and allow the mixture to cool to 140°F (60°C). A temperature above that can compromise the preservative.
5. Add the essential oils and preservative, and blend for 5 to 10 seconds more.
6. Pour or spoon the mixture into tins or glass jars and allow it to cool and thicken before capping them.

HOW TO USE

Massage into your chest at bedtime or anytime you want to ease congestion.

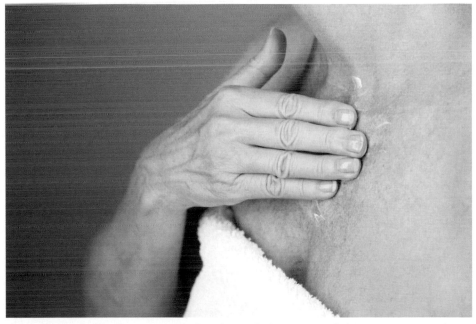

The combination of soothing essential oils and a gentle chest massage helps to open up your chest and airways.

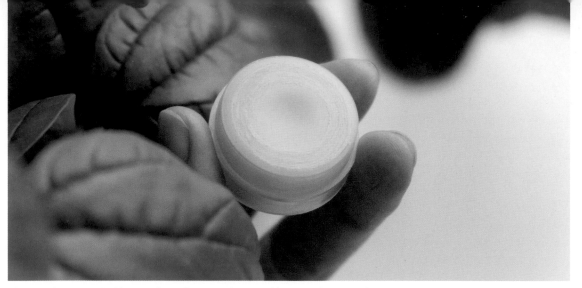

Chamomile essential oil helps relieve the pain of chapped lips, but the scent also provides a sense of well-being.

CHAPPED LIP SALVE
MAKES 2 OUNCES (60ML)

Hydrating mango butter, coconut oil, jojoba, and calendula oil create a powerful foundation to heal and nurture chapped lips, with the essential oils of frankincense and chamomile offering their anti-inflammatory and skin-soothing properties for added protection.

EQUIPMENT

- 2-ounce (60ml) metal tin, glass jar, or multiple lip balm tubes
- Small glass measuring cup
- Measuring spoons
- Glass pipettes
- Wooden stir stick

INGREDIENTS

Base:
- 1 teaspoon (5ml) mango butter
- 1 tablespoon (5g) candelilla wax
- 1 tablespoon (15ml) coconut oil
- 1 tablespoon (15ml) calendula oil
- 1 tablespoon (15ml) jojoba
- 6 drops vitamin E, optional

Essential Oils:
- ¼ teaspoon (1.25ml) frankincense
- 4 drops chamomile
- 3 drops yarrow

HOW TO MAKE

1. Melt the butter, wax, and base oils in the measuring cup in the microwave, 15 seconds at a time, stopping to stir with your stir stick in between.
2. Once fully melted, add the vitamin E (if using) and essential oils. Stir to blend.
3. Pour carefully into containers as the liquid will be hot.
4. Leave for 1 to 2 hours until fully solidified before capping and labeling.

HOW TO USE

Massage into dry, chapped, or irritated lips to sooth and protect.

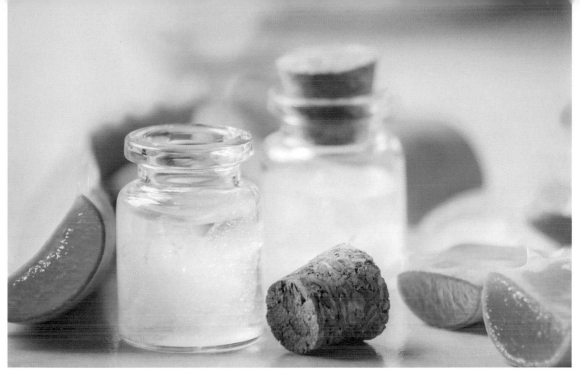

This hand sanitizer works well and, unlike many commercial hand sanitizers, it smells fantastic.

EUCALYPTUS LIME HAND SANITIZER
MAKES 8 OUNCES (250ML)

I carry this fresh and vibrant sanitizer in my purse to have available when I'm traveling or simply out and about and wanting to stay germ-free. Lime is a powerful antibacterial essential oil, and eucalyptus offers immunity support and virus protection.

EQUIPMENT
- Measuring cup
- Measuring spoons
- Pump or squeeze bottle
- Glass pipettes
- Funnel

INGREDIENTS
Base:
- $\frac{2}{3}$ cup (160ml) isopropyl alcohol
- $\frac{1}{3}$ cup (80ml) aloe vera liquid

Essential Oils:
- $\frac{1}{2}$ teaspoon (2.5ml) lime
- 12 drops eucalyptus

HOW TO MAKE
1. Measure and pour the alcohol and aloe vera liquid into the bottle using the funnel.
2. Add the essential oils to the bottle and swirl to incorporate. Cap.

HOW TO USE
Pour about $\frac{1}{2}$ teaspoon (2.5ml) into the palm of one hand and then massage all over both hands, especially on your fingertips.

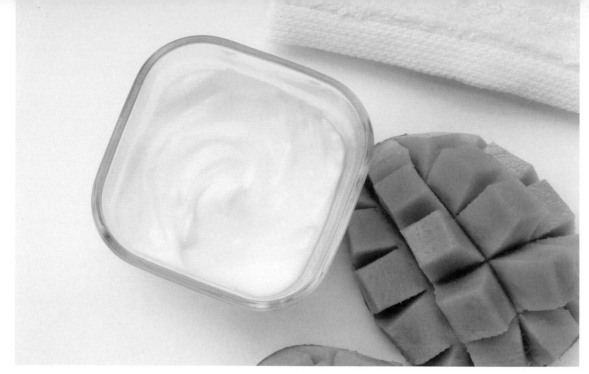

Pamper your fingers and toes before grooming to keep them in tip-top shape.

CUTICLE AND CALLUS SOFTENER
MAKES 4 OUNCES (125ML)

Taking time to do our own grooming rather than spending hours—and dollars—paying others to do it can feel like a self-nurturing treat. Use this cream to soften your cuticles and calluses for an at-home spa-quality mani-pedi. Luscious skin softeners like aloe vera, mango butter, and coconut oil prepare your hands for a manicure and your feet for some serious scrubbing, leaving them soft and callus-free. *See Emulsion Tips on page 67.*

EQUIPMENT
- Small glass bowl
- Glass measuring cup
- Thermometer, optional
- 4-ounce (125ml) glass jar or tin
- Double boiler, optional

INGREDIENTS

Water Phase:
- ¼ cup (60ml) lavender hydrosol or distilled water
- 2 tablespoons (30ml) aloe vera gel
- ⅛ teaspoon (0.5ml) citric acid

Oil Phase:
- 2 tablespoons (30ml) mango butter
- 2 tablespoons (11g) e-wax
- 1 tablespoon (15ml) coconut oil
- 1 tablespoon (15ml) jojoba

Essential Oils:
- ½ teaspoon (2.5ml) lavender
- 6 drops neroli, optional

Preservative:
- ½ teaspoon (2.5ml) Germaben II

HOW TO MAKE

Prepare the Water Phase

1. Combine water phase ingredients in a glass bowl and heat in the microwave for 1 minute until the citric acid is dissolved.
2. Stir and test the temperature with your thermometer. If it's not yet at 160°F–170°F (71°–77°C), microwave for 1 more minute and then set it aside.

Prepare the Oil Phase

1. Melt all the oil phase ingredients in a double boiler (or in the microwave, 1 minute at a time, stirring in between). Stir until all the butters are melted.
2. Heat to the same temperature as the water phase, letting cool if needed to reach the correct temperature range.

Blend the Phases

1. When phases are within the correct temperature range and are approximately the same temperature, pour the water phase into the small blender.
2. Add the oil phase—it should immediately turn white.
3. Blend for 5 to 10 seconds until fully combined.
4. Open the blender and allow the mixture to cool to 140°F (60°C). A temperature above that can compromise the preservative.
5. Add the essential oils and preservative, and blend for 5 to 10 seconds more.
6. Pour or spoon the mixture into tins or glass jars and allow it to cool and thicken before capping them.

HOW TO USE

Massage into your heels before exfoliating with a callus remover tool or pumice stone and dab a bit on your cuticles to soften them before trimming.

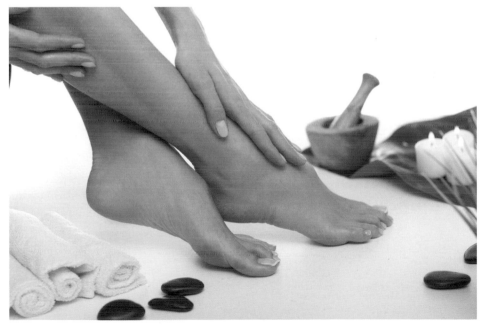

Begin your next manicure and pedicure with this soothing emulsion.

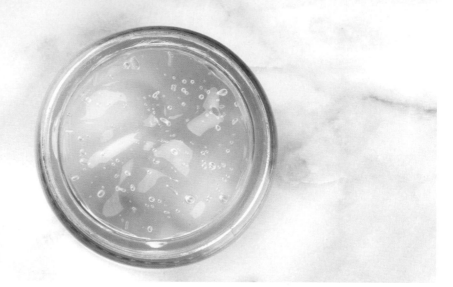

This antiseptic keeps well in the refrigerator or even the freezer, to naturally treat minor cuts and abrasions when needed.

ALOE ANTISEPTIC WIPE
MAKES 1 OUNCE (30ML)

Lavender, eucalyptus, and aloe vera are all antifungal, antimicrobial, infection-fighting, and skin-healing, creating an all-natural treatment for minor cuts and abrasions. Keep a small container in the freezer to pull out as needed.

EQUIPMENT

- 1-ounce (30ml) tin or jar
- Measuring spoons
- Wooden stir stick

INGREDIENTS

Base:
- 1 tablespoon (15ml) aloe vera gel
- 1 tablespoon (15ml) witch hazel

Essential Oils:
- 22 drops lavender
- 8 drops eucalyptus

HOW TO MAKE

1. Add the aloe vera and witch hazel to the container.
2. Drop in the essential oils.
3. Stir with the stir stick and cap.

HOW TO USE

Dip a cotton swab or pad into the antiseptic and gently dab it on the wound before covering it with a clean dressing. Store in the refrigerator or freezer if you're making enough to save for multiple uses.

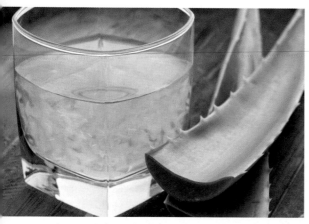

Aloe vera helps to heal your skin and fight infections.

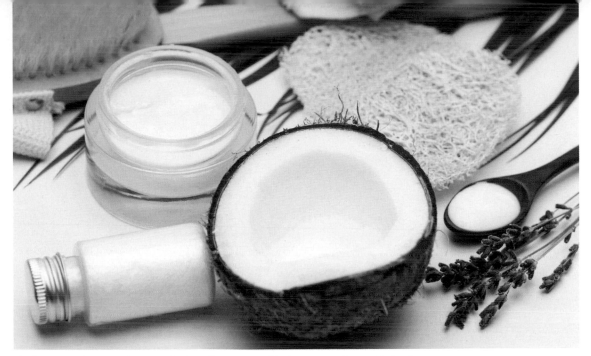

The base ingredients and essential oils in this cream will help promote faster skin healing.

SHAVING NICK SOOTHER

MAKES 2 OUNCES (60ML)

Harness the power of healing essential oils to instantly move small nicks and cuts into the healing phase.

EQUIPMENT
- Small glass measuring cup
- Measuring spoons
- Wooden stir stick
- 2-ounce (60ml) tin or jar
- Double boiler, optional

INGREDIENTS
Base:
- 1 tablespoon (5g) candelilla wax
- 1 tablespoon (30ml) mango butter or shea butter
- 1 tablespoon (30ml) virgin coconut oil
- 1 teaspoon (5ml) aloe vera gel
- 1 teaspoon (5ml) glycerin

Essential Oils:
- ¼ teaspoon (1.25ml) lavender
- 6 drops tea tree

HOW TO MAKE
1. If using shea butter, use a double boiler to melt and hold at temperature for 20 minutes to avoid crystallization of product later.
2. Melt the wax, coconut oil, and butter (if not yet melted) in the microwave for 30 seconds. Stir until all the pieces are fully dissolved.
3. Add the aloe vera gel, glycerin, and essential oils. Stir to incorporate.
4. Pour into the tin or jar and let sit for 1 hour before capping.
5. Let sit for 2 hours or overnight to solidify before first use.

HOW TO USE
Dab onto small nicks to soothe and support healing. Keep indoors (your medicine cabinet is the perfect place) as this soother can melt at high temperatures.

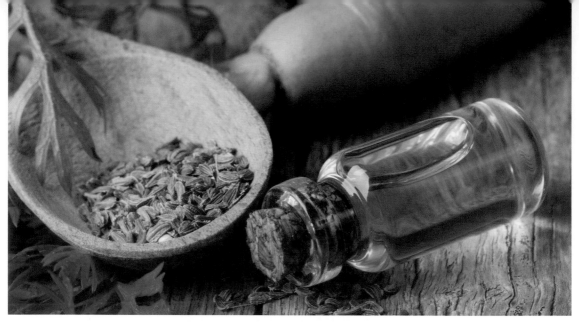

Carrot seed oil is included in this salve for its soothing and healing properties.

WOUND-HEALING SALVE

MAKES 2 OUNCES (60ML)

The magic of this salve comes first from the base oils: calendula, arnica, carrot seed, and camellia tea seed oil are all known for their skin-soothing properties. Lavender offers additional treatment, gently detoxifying the skin and preparing it for healing.

EQUIPMENT

- One 2-ounce (60ml) metal tin or two 1-ounce (30ml) metal tins
- Small glass measuring cup
- Wooden stir stick

INGREDIENTS

Base:

- 1 tablespoon (5g) candelilla wax
- 1 tablespoon (15ml) calendula oil
- 1 tablespoon (15ml) arnica oil
- 1 tablespoon (15ml) camellia tea seed oil
- 1 tablespoon (15ml) jojoba
- 1 teaspoon (5ml) carrot seed oil

Essential Oils:

- ¼ teaspoon (1.25ml) lavender
- ⅛ teaspoon (0.5 ml) frankincense
- 3 drops helichrysum

HOW TO MAKE

1. Melt the wax and base oils in the measuring cup in the microwave, 15 seconds at a time, stopping to stir with stir stick in between.
2. Once the mixture is fully melted, add the essential oils and stir to blend.
3. Pour carefully into the tin as the liquid will be hot.
4. Leave for 1 to 2 hours or until fully solidified before capping and labeling.

HOW TO USE

Massage into minor cuts and scrapes to facilitate natural healing.

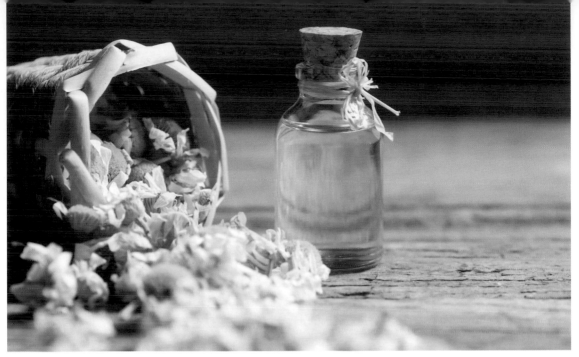

This balm combines chamomile oil with chamomile essential oil to calm inflamed skin and prevent further irritation.

CHAMOMILE BURN BALM
MAKES 2 OUNCES (60ML)

Minor burns are unavoidable as we cook, bake, or otherwise "play" with fire, and chamomile is known for its powerful anti-inflammatory and calming properties. I keep this balm handy to apply immediately when needed, as quick topical application prevents more severe irritation of the skin.

EQUIPMENT
- 2-ounce (60ml) metal tin or glass jar
- Small glass measuring cup
- Wooden stir stick

INGREDIENTS
Base:
- 2 tablespoons (30ml) chamomile oil
- 1 tablespoon (15ml) coconut oil
- 1 tablespoon (15ml) shea butter or mango butter
- 1 tablespoon (5g) candelilla wax

Essential Oils:
- ⅛ teaspoon (0.5 ml) lavender
- 8 drops eucalyptus
- 3 drops chamomile

HOW TO MAKE
1. Melt the base ingredients in the measuring cup in the microwave, 15 seconds at a time, stopping to stir with stir stick in between.
2. Once fully melted, add the essential oils. Stir to blend.
3. Pour carefully into the tin as the liquid will be hot.
4. Leave for 1 to 2 hours or until fully solidified before capping and labeling.

HOW TO USE
Massage into minor cuts, scrapes, or wounds to facilitate natural healing.

Bath salts are easy to make and quickly elevate a simple bath to a luxurious, pampering experience.

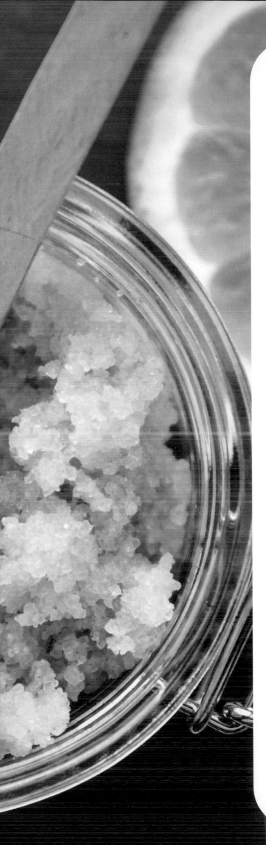

HOME SPA RECIPES

Taking a moment to nurture, nourish, and restore yourself is not a privilege, it's essential in today's world of stimulation overload and challenging world events. Unplugging and letting yourself just "be" using beautifully scented and sensual products is a way to anchor yourself and reset in between busy weekdays, at the end of every day, or as a monthly ritual—whatever your life allows. Essential oils induce healing, health, and happiness by working in synergy with our own physiology. Bring the flowers and forest inside, simply and naturally, to restore your sense of balance and equanimity anytime life calls for it. These are some of the simplest products to make and they pay big dividends when used consistently to recalibrate your mind and body.

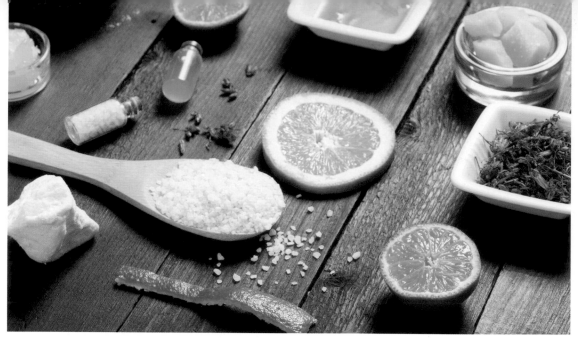

These bath salts soften your skin and lighten your mood.

TANGERINE CALENDULA BATH SALTS
MAKES 8 OUNCES (250ML)

Bath salts induce a moment of pause and a retreat from the world, and this salt blend that includes both citrus and flowers allows for a healing and healthy soak. Tangerine essential oil has an uplifting, sweet aroma and an antibacterial, calming chemical profile. Calendula flower petals are delicate and easily dissolve in bath water, while softening your skin.

EQUIPMENT
- Mixing bowl
- Stirring spoon
- Measuring cups
- Measuring spoons
- Glass jar or bottle
- Funnel, if using bottle

INGREDIENTS
Base:
- 1 cup (250ml) sea salt
- ¼ cup (60ml) calendula flower petals
- 1 teaspoon (5ml) pink clay

Essential Oil:
- 1 tablespoon (15ml) tangerine

HOW TO MAKE
1. Add the salt to the bowl and drizzle the clay and essential oil over them. Stir to fully combine.
2. Add the calendula flowers and stir gently to incorporate.
3. Transfer to a jar or into a bottle using the funnel. Let sit overnight to allow the salts to fully absorb the essential oil.

HOW TO USE
Pour ¼ cup (60ml) into running bath water. Soak and enjoy!

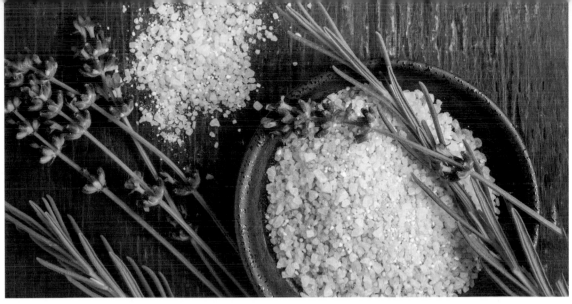

These bath salts are perfect for adding a luxurious, relaxing bath to your pre-bedtime routine.

PURE LAVENDER BATH SALTS
MAKES 8 OUNCES (250ML)

Nothing beats lavender for its sedative effects, so it's the perfect marriage with bath salts. Enjoy its calming and pain-relieving effects as you give yourself a lavender retreat. Lavender petals add beauty to the salts and make a great addition when giving these as a gift but are optional (and will need to be rinsed down the drain after your bath).

EQUIPMENT
- Mixing bowl
- Stirring spoon
- Measuring cup
- Measuring spoons
- Glass jar or bottle
- Funnel, if using bottle

INGREDIENTS
Base:
- 8 ounces (250ml) sea salt
- 1 tablespoon (15ml) lavender petals, optional for decoration
- 1 teaspoon (5ml) lavender mica, optional for color

Essential Oil:
- 1 tablespoon (15ml) lavender essential oil

HOW TO MAKE
1. Add the salt to the bowl and spoon the mica (if using) over them. Stir to fully combine into one light lavender color.
2. Add the essential oil and stir to combine.
3. Add the lavender petals (if using) and stir gently to incorporate.
4. Transfer to a glass jar or bottle, using a funnel. Allow to sit overnight so the salts fully absorb the lavender essential oil.

HOW TO USE
Pour ¼ cup (60ml) into running bath water. Soak and enjoy!

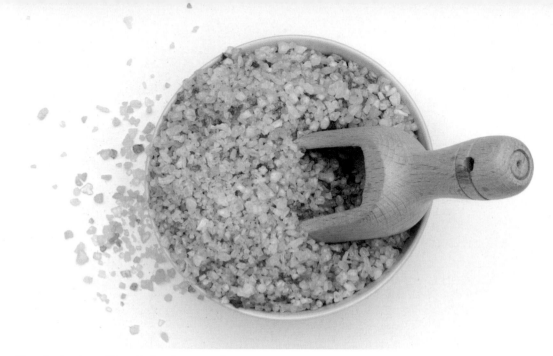

These bath salts uplift and help relieve muscle pain.

PINK GRAPEFRUIT BATH SALTS
MAKES 8 OUNCES (250ML)

Pink grapefruit might be my favorite essential oil, because of its fresh and versatile nature. It blends well with florals and wood scents, but also stands up well on its own with a sweet and light aroma that is ever-pleasing. Its chemical profile is uplifting, calming, and supportive of the immune system, and it acts as a tonic, decongestant, and pain reliever. That's a lot packed into one sweet treat!

EQUIPMENT
- Mixing bowl
- Stirring spoon
- Measuring cup
- Measuring spoons
- Glass jars

INGREDIENTS
Base:
- 8 ounces (250ml) pink or white sea salt
- 1 tablespoon (15ml) fresh grapefruit zest

Essential Oil:
- 1 tablespoon (15ml) pink grapefruit

HOW TO MAKE
1. Add the salt to the mixing bowl and drizzle the zest and essential oil over the top. Stir to fully combine. Adjust the scent by using a bit more essential oil, if desired—pink grapefruit is light and volatile, so I often use a bit more of it to get to my desired scent level.
2. Transfer to glass jars. Allow to sit overnight to fully incorporate the scent.

HOW TO USE
Pour ¼ cup (60ml) into running bath water. Soak and enjoy!

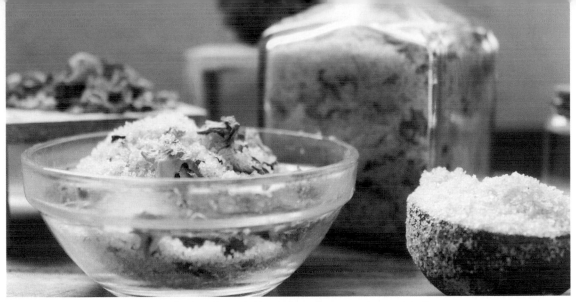

This is forest bathing at its finest—a floral and woody blend of salt, flowers, and essential oil.

CYPRESS ROSE BATH SALTS
MAKES 8 OUNCES (250ML)

Retreat into a soothing sanctuary with this combination of rose and pine—a protective and grounding blend that heals the heart and calms the mind. Let this gorgeous forest aroma take you deep into the woods as you close your eyes and breathe in the naturally therapeutic essential oils from two of the most widely used and popular plants in the world. Cypress essential oil reduces inflammation and boosts the immune system, while rose is known to mitigate anxiety, stress, depression, and pain.

EQUIPMENT
- Mixing bowl
- Stirring spoon
- Measuring cup
- Measuring spoons
- Glass jars or bottle
- Funnel, if using bottle

INGREDIENTS
Base:
- 1 cup (250ml) pink salt
- ¼ cup (60ml) dried rose petals

Essential Oils:
- 1 tablespoon (15ml) rose in jojoba or 1 teaspoon (5ml) rose otto
- 1 teaspoon (5ml) cypress

HOW TO MAKE
1. Add salt to the bowl and drizzle the rose in jojoba or rose otto essential oil and white pine essential oil over them. Stir to combine.
2. Add the dried rose petals and stir to incorporate.
3. Transfer to a glass jar or bottle, using a funnel if placing in a bottle.

HOW TO USE
Pour ¼ cup (60ml) into running bath water. Soak and enjoy!

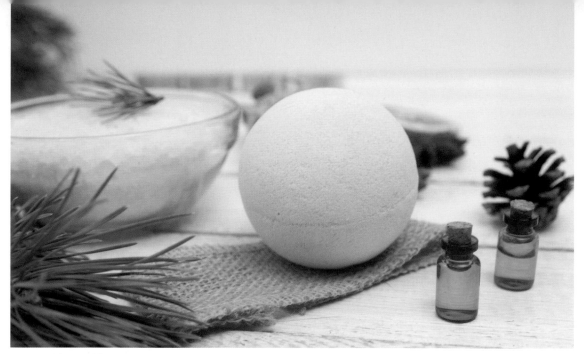

Fresh and foresty, black spruce is one of the most delightful wood essential oils.

BLACK SPRUCE BATH BOMBS
MAKES 8 MEDIUM BATH BOMBS

Black spruce is a natural pain reliever, grounding the nervous system and helping to alleviate respiratory issues. It's one of my favorite aromas, instantly transporting me to an enchanted forest; it makes a wonderful addition to your bath paraphernalia. Deeply inhaling the pure scent of a spruce forest will leave you feeling rejuvenated, restored, and ready for life's next challenge.

EQUIPMENT
- Mixing bowl
- Stirring spoon
- Measuring cup
- Measuring spoons
- Bath bomb molds

INGREDIENTS
Dry:
- 1 cup (250ml) baking soda
- ½ cup (125ml) citric acid
- ½ cup (125ml) Epsom salt
- ½ cup (125ml) cornstarch or arrowroot powder
- ½–1 teaspoon (2.5–5ml) spirulina, optional for color

Wet:
- 3 tablespoons (45ml) melted coconut oil
- 2 tablespoons (30ml) sunflower oil
- 1 tablespoon (15ml) water

Essential Oil:
- ¼ teaspoon (1.25ml) black spruce

HOW TO MAKE

1. Mix the dry ingredients together to incorporate. Press out all the clumps with the back of the spoon until the mixture is smooth and the desired color (if using spirulina) is achieved.

2. Mix together the wet ingredients and the essential oil and stir to incorporate.

3. **Slowly** pour the wet ingredients into the dry, and **slowly** stir the mixture while you pour. There will be some fizzing from the water, but by pouring and stirring slowly you can minimize it. (Stirring too quickly sets off the "bomb" reaction—you want to save that for the bath!)

4. Stir until everything is fully incorporated and the mixture sticks together. If the mix seems too dry or powdery, add a bit more oil or spray with water until the mixture gently sticks together. If the mixture seems too wet, add a bit more arrowroot powder or cornstarch, until the consistency is like a very dry dough.

5. Spoon the mixture into each half of the mold until slightly rounded/overfull and then press the two mold halves firmly together and hold for a moment to tighten. Ideally none of the mixture will spill out and the sides of the mold will touch and close completely, but if a bit extends outside the edges, that is fine.

6. Let stand 1 to 5 minutes before unmolding by gently and slowly twisting the sides in opposite directions. Be patient and careful!

7. Holding the bath bombs very loosely, gently place them one by one onto wax paper or a plate and let dry for 24 to 48 hours before handling or using. They need to dry to firm up and be ready for handling without breaking.

HOW TO USE

Drop into the bathwater as your tub fills. Enjoy the fizz either before you get in or while you're soaking. Breathe deeply and take in the healing, heavenly aroma to restore and relax.

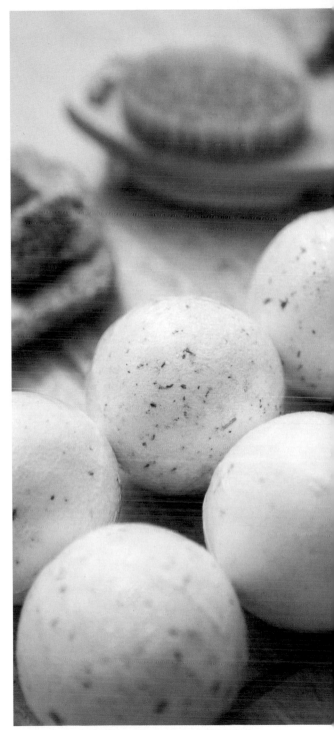

These restorative bath bombs are thoughtful gifts for family members and friends.

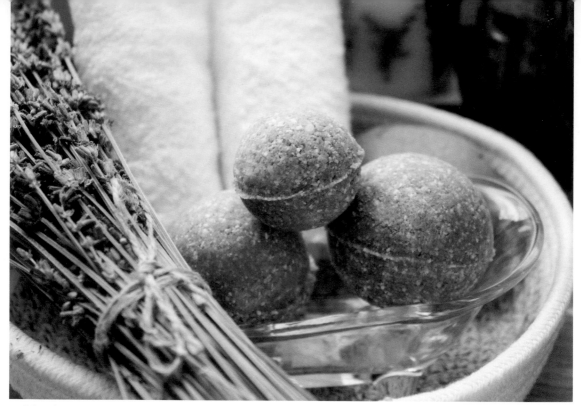

Bath bombs are easy to make with a bit of time and patience, and they create a fun and fizzy bath experience.

LAVENDER FIELDS BATH BOMBS
MAKES 8 MEDIUM BATH BOMBS

For lavender purists, this transportive bomb takes you to southern France where the lavender fields are endless and vast, reaching the horizon. It's the quintessential balancing oil, and this explosive little bomb will eradicate all your cares and worries.

EQUIPMENT
- Mixing bowl
- Stirring spoon
- Measuring cup
- Measuring spoons
- Bath bomb molds

INGREDIENTS
Dry:
- 1 cup (250ml) baking soda
- ½ cup (125ml) citric acid
- ½ cup (125ml) Epsom salt
- ½ cup (125ml) cornstarch or arrowroot powder

Wet:
- 3 tablespoons (45ml) melted coconut oil
- 2 tablespoons (30ml) sunflower oil
- 1 tablespoon (15ml) water

Essential Oil:
- ¼ teaspoon (1.25ml) lavender

HOW TO MAKE

1. Mix the dry ingredients together to incorporate. Press out all the clumps with the back of the spoon until the mixture is smooth and the desired color is achieved.

2. Mix together the wet ingredients and the essential oil and stir to incorporate.

3. **Slowly** pour the wet ingredients into the dry, and **slowly** stir the mixture while you pour. There will be some fizzing from the water, but by pouring and stirring slowly you can minimize it. (Stirring too quickly sets off the "bomb" reaction—you want to save that for the bath!)

4. Stir until everything is fully incorporated and the mixture sticks together. If the mix seems too dry or powdery, add a bit more oil or spray with water until the mixture gently sticks together. If the mixture seems too wet, add a bit more arrowroot powder or cornstarch, until the consistency is like a very dry dough.

5. Spoon the mixture into each half of the mold until slightly rounded/overfull and then press the two mold halves firmly together and hold for a moment to tighten. Ideally none of the mixture will spill out and the sides of the mold will touch and close completely, but if a bit extends outside the edges, that is fine.

6. Let stand 1 to 5 minutes before unmolding by gently and slowly twisting the sides in opposite directions. Be patient and careful!

7. Holding the bath bombs very loosely, gently place them one by one onto wax paper or a plate and let dry for 24 to 48 hours before handling or using. They need to dry to firm up and be ready for handling without breaking.

HOW TO USE

Drop into the bathwater as your tub fills. Enjoy the fizz either before you get in or while you're soaking. Breathe deeply and take in the healing, heavenly aroma to restore and relax.

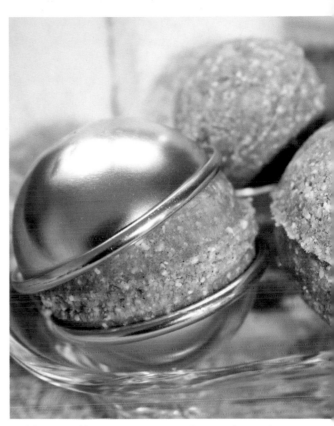

Bath bomb molds come in many sizes, for your choice of fizz level in your bath.

TIP: If you want perfect, uniform color rather than a rustic, mottled color, try pressing out each dry ingredient before mixing.

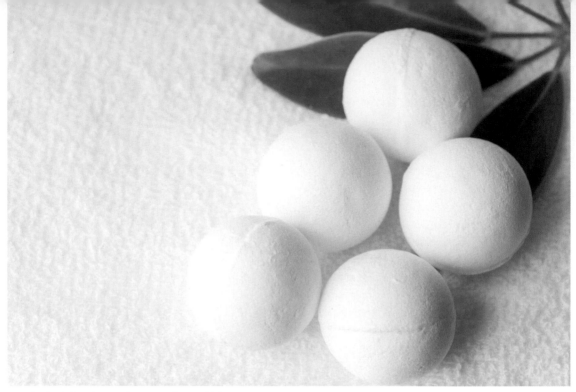

Use this bath bomb to soften your skin and lift your mood.

LEMON VERBENA BATH BOMBS
MAKES 8 MEDIUM BATH BOMBS

Lemon verbena is noted for easing cramps, indigestion, low mood, and anxiety. Relieve any tension your body contains with this invigorating bath bomb that will have you swooning with its vibrant and incomparably fresh aroma.

EQUIPMENT

- Mixing bowl
- Stirring spoon
- Measuring cup
- Measuring spoons
- Bath bomb molds

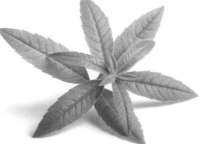

INGREDIENTS
Dry:

- 1 cup (250ml) baking soda
- ½ cup (125ml) citric acid
- ½ cup (125ml) Epsom salt
- ½ cup (125ml) cornstarch or arrowroot powder

Wet:

- 3 tablespoons (45ml) melted coconut oil
- 2 tablespoons (30ml) sunflower oil
- 1 tablespoon (15ml) water

Essential Oil:

- ¼ teaspoon (1.25ml) lemon verbena

HOW TO MAKE

1. Mix the dry ingredients together to incorporate. Press out all the clumps with the back of the spoon until the mixture is smooth and the desired color is achieved.
2. Mix together the wet ingredients and the essential oil and stir to incorporate.
3. **Slowly** pour the wet ingredients into the dry, and **slowly** stir the mixture while you pour. There will be some fizzing from the water, but by pouring and stirring slowly you can minimize it. (Stirring too quickly sets off the "bomb" reaction—you want to save that for the bath!)
4. Stir until everything is fully incorporated and the mixture sticks together. If the mix seems too dry or powdery, add a bit more oil or spray with water until the mixture gently sticks together. If the mixture seems too wet, add a bit more arrowroot powder or cornstarch, until the consistency is like a very dry dough.
5. Spoon the mixture into each half of the mold until slightly rounded/overfull and then press the two mold halves firmly together and hold for a moment to tighten. Ideally none of the mixture will spill out and the sides of the mold will touch and close completely, but if a bit extends outside the edges, that is fine.
6. Let stand 1 to 5 minutes before unmolding by gently and slowly twisting the sides in opposite directions. Be patient and careful!
7. Holding the bath bombs very loosely, gently place them one by one onto wax paper or a plate and let dry for 24 to 48 hours before handling or using. They need to dry to firm up and be ready for handling without breaking.

HOW TO USE

Drop into the bathwater as your tub fills. Enjoy the fizz either before you get in or while you're soaking. Breathe deeply and take in the healing, heavenly aroma to restore and relax.

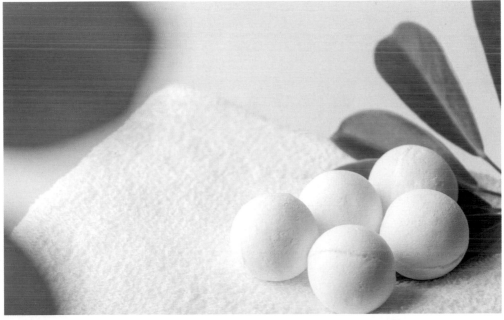

These bath bombs will help to ease tension and anxiety, indigestion, and cramps, while also lifting your spirits.

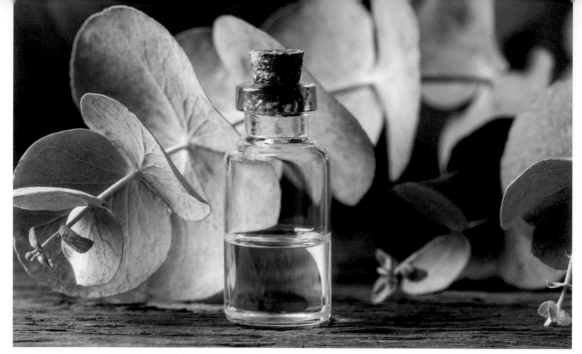

Eucalyptus essential oil adds a refreshing balance to the soothing rose scent.

EUCALYPTUS ROSE BATH OIL
MAKES 8 OUNCES (250ML)

Baths are one of the best ways to ground our energy and bring us home to ourselves. This pampering blend of eucalyptus and rose creates a spa-worthy ambience any time to you need to relax and restore.

EQUIPMENT
- Glass bottle
- Funnel
- Measuring spoons
- Pipettes

INGREDIENTS
Base:
- 8 ounces (250ml) carrier oil or a combination of carrier oils, such as avocado, peach kernel, and sunflower

Essential Oils:
- 1 tablespoon (15ml) rose in jojoba or ¼ teaspoon (1.25ml) rose otto
- ½ teaspoon (2.5ml) eucalyptus

HOW TO MAKE
1. Fill your bottle with your chosen carrier oil or carrier oil mixture, leaving a bit of space at the top.
2. Using a clean pipette for each essential oil, add the essential oils.
3. Cap and gently swirl to incorporate. Adjust scent to preference, if needed.

HOW TO USE
Add approximately 2 tablespoons (30ml) to running bath water and soak. Luxuriate in the hydrating, softening water and breathe deeply to relax and restore.

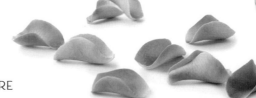

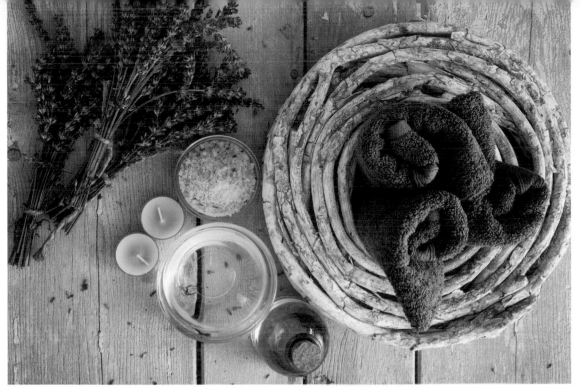

This woodsy, relaxing oil is perfect for any time you need a moment of deep relaxation.

LAVENDER FOREST BATH OIL
MAKES 8 OUNCES (250ML)

Lavender lovers will find nirvana in this divine blend, which transports us to a gentle forest where we can close our eyes, breathe deeply, and immerse ourselves in twilight dreams.

EQUIPMENT
- Glass bottle
- Measuring spoons
- Funnel
- Pipettes

INGREDIENTS
Base:
- 8 ounces (250ml) carrier oil or a combination of carrier oils
- **Essential Oils:**
- 2 teaspoons (10ml) lavender
- 1 teaspoon (5ml) spruce, pine, or cypress

HOW TO MAKE
1. Fill your bottle with your chosen carrier oil or carrier oil mixture, leaving a bit of space at the top.
2. Using a clean pipette for each essential oil, add the essential oils.
3. Cap and gently swirl to incorporate. Adjust scent to preference, if needed.

HOW TO USE
Add approximately 2 tablespoons (30ml) to running bath water and soak. Luxuriate in the hydrating, softening water and breathe deeply to relax and restore.

NEROLI ORANGE BATH OIL
MAKES 8 OUNCES (250ML)

Neroli from bitter orange tree flowers is a premium oil, but worth the splurge for a small amount in order to create an upscale bath blend. It reduces pain and inflammation, and smells heavenly when matched with its vibrant cousin, sweet orange.

EQUIPMENT
- Glass bottle
- Funnel
- Measuring spoons
- Pipettes

INGREDIENTS
Base:
- 8 ounces (250ml) carrier oil or a combination of carrier oils

Essential Oils:
- 2 teaspoons (10ml) sweet orange
- 1 teaspoon (5ml) bergamot
- 6 drops neroli

HOW TO MAKE
1. Fill your bottle with your chosen carrier oil or carrier oil mixture, leaving a bit of space at the top.
2. Using a clean pipette for each essential oil, add the essential oils.
3. Cap and gently swirl to incorporate. Adjust scent to preference, if needed.

HOW TO USE
Add approximately 2 tablespoons (30ml) to running bath water and soak. Luxuriate in the hydrating, softening water and breathe deeply to relax and restore.

CEDARWOOD SAGE BATH OIL
MAKES 8 OUNCES (250ML)

Sage essential oil helps ease muscle and joint pain and eliminates toxins from the body, while cedarwood offers a woody aromatic counterpoint with natural sedative properties.

EQUIPMENT
- Glass bottle
- Funnel
- Measuring spoons
- Pipettes

INGREDIENTS
Base:
- 8 ounces (250ml) carrier oil or a combination of carrier oils

Essential Oils:
- ¼ teaspoon (1.25ml) cedarwood
- ¼ teaspoon (1.25ml) sage
- 1 teaspoon (5ml) sweet orange

HOW TO MAKE
1. Fill your bottle with your chosen carrier oil or carrier oil mixture, leaving a bit of space at the top.
2. Using a clean pipette for each essential oil, add the essential oils.
3. Cap and gently swirl to incorporate. Adjust scent to preference, if needed.

HOW TO USE
Add approximately 2 tablespoons (30ml) to running bath water and soak. Luxuriate in the hydrating, softening water and breathe deeply to relax and restore.

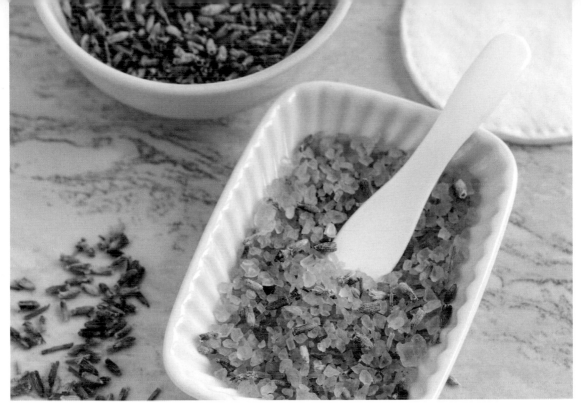

There are few things as luxurious and relaxing as a salt soak after a long day on your feet.

LAVENDER LIME FOOT SOAK
MAKES 8 OUNCES (250ML)

After a long day, soothe tired feet with an easily assembled foot soak. The lavender-lime blend is skin-healing and calming.

EQUIPMENT
- Mixing bowl
- Stirring spoon
- Glass measuring cup
- Measuring spoons
- Glass jar

INGREDIENTS
Base:
- 8 ounces (250ml) Epsom salt

Essential Oils:
- 1 tablespoon (15ml) lavender
- 1 teaspoon (5ml) lime

HOW TO MAKE
1. Add the Epsom salt to a large bowl.
2. Pour the essential oils over the salt. Stir thoroughly to blend.
3. Transfer to a jar and allow to infuse overnight before using.

HOW TO USE
Measure ¼ cup (60ml) into a tub of very warm water and soak your feet to restore and rejuvenate.

PEPPERMINT MANDARIN FOOT SOAK
MAKES 8 OUNCES (250ML)

After a long day, soothe tired feet with an easily assembled foot soak. This soak is an invigorating and restorative treat.

EQUIPMENT

- Mixing bowl
- Stirring spoon
- Glass measuring cup
- Measuring spoons
- Glass jar

INGREDIENTS
Base:
- 8 ounces (250ml) Epsom salt

Essential Oils:
- 1 tablespoon (15ml) mandarin
- ¼ teaspoon (1.25ml) peppermint

HOW TO MAKE

1. Add the Epsom salt to a large bowl.
2. Pour the essential oils over the salt. Stir thoroughly to blend.
3. Transfer to a jar and allow to infuse overnight before using.

HOW TO USE

Measure ¼ cup (60ml) into a tub of very warm water and soak your feet to restore and rejuvenate.

CYPRESS FOREST BODY OIL
MAKES 8 OUNCES (250ML)

Massage oils are an easy treat to whip up anytime the mood strikes. Luxuriate in soothing oils for skin, muscle, and mood health while giving or receiving a loving massage. Use all over or just on your feet, hands and ears for a qigong-inspired daily self-massage that invigorates the internal organs for optimal health. Daily self-massage stimulates our lymphatic system, increases circulation, helps the body detox, and improves sleep, so don't wait for someone else to do it—take these healthy delights into your own hands!

EQUIPMENT

- Glass bottle
- Funnel
- Glass measuring cup
- Measuring spoons

INGREDIENTS
Carrier Oils:
- 4 ounces (125ml) avocado oil
- 2 ounces (60ml) sunflower seed oil
- 1 ounce (30ml) apricot kernel oil
- 1 ounce (30ml) arnica oil
- ¼ teaspoon (1.25ml) vitamin E oil

Essential Oils:
- 1 teaspoon (5ml) cypress
- ¼ teaspoon (1.25ml) white pine
- ¼ teaspoon (1.25ml) juniper berry

HOW TO MAKE

1. Add the carrier oils to a bottle with the funnel.
2. Add the essential oils.
3. Cap and gently swirl to incorporate.

HOW TO USE

Use this allover massage oil for general release and relaxation.

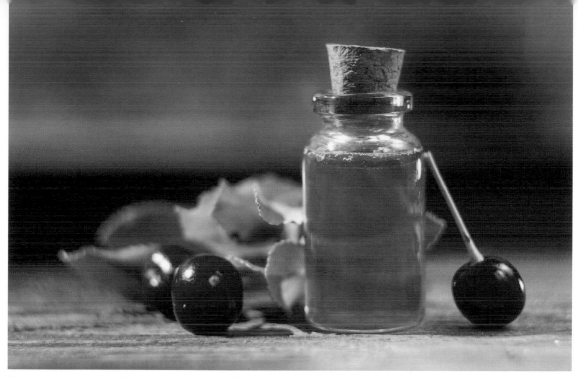

These beneficial oils combine to create a powerful massaging oil to treat your most sensitive skin.

BREAST AND DÉCOLLETAGE OIL
MAKES 8 OUNCES (250ML)

To hydrate and protect the delicate décolletage, breast, and neck areas, use this warming and healing massage oil.

EQUIPMENT
- Glass bottle
- Funnel
- Glass measuring cup
- Measuring spoons

INGREDIENTS
Carrier Oils:
- 4 ounces (125ml) almond oil
- 3 ounces (90ml) calendula oil
- 1 tablespoon (15ml) cherry seed oil
- 1 teaspoon (5ml) argan oil
- 1 teaspoon (5ml) vitamin E oil

Essential Oil:
- 1 teaspoon (5ml) rose in jojoba

HOW TO MAKE
1. Add the carrier oils to a bottle with the funnel.
2. Add the essential oils.
3. Cap and gently swirl to incorporate.

HOW TO USE
Massage into your chest and neck areas daily or as desired to hydrate and keep your skin soft, smooth, and moisturized.

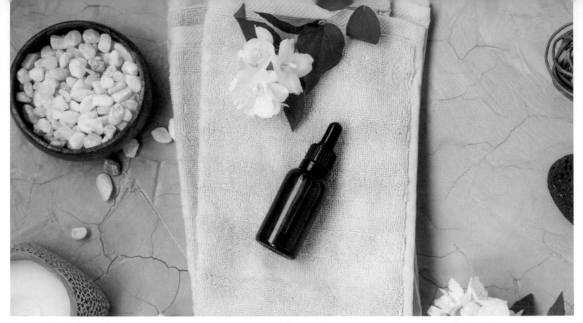

A smooth oil with sensual aromatics is a great way to set the stage for connection, or simply to delight the senses.

JASMINE APHRODISIAC OIL
MAKES 8 OUNCES (250ML)

Heating up the mood is easy with this floral-filled, sultry, jasmine-infused body oil to trade massages and sensual pleasures. The carrier oils contain a plethora of vitamins, minerals, and antioxidants that hydrate, heal, and restore elasticity while the jasmine essential oil opens the heart and offers a dreamy, sensual boost.

EQUIPMENT

- Glass bottle
- Funnel
- Glass measuring cup
- Measuring spoons

INGREDIENTS
Carrier Oils:

- 2 ounces (60ml) pomegranate seed oil
- 2 ounces (60ml) sunflower seed oil
- 2 ounces (60ml) avocado oil
- 1 tablespoon (15ml) strawberry seed oil
- 1 tablespoon (15ml) watermelon seed oil
- 1 tablespoon (15ml) cherry seed oil
- 1 tablespoon (15ml) jasmine-infused jojoba
- 1 teaspoon (5ml) vanilla-infused jojoba
- 12 drops vitamin E oil

HOW TO MAKE

1. Add the carrier oils to a bottle with the funnel.
2. Cap and gently swirl to incorporate.

HOW TO USE

Use this allover massage oil for a sensual boost.

TIP: If you can't find the infused jojobas, use regular jojoba and ½ teaspoon (2.5ml) of jasmine absolute and ⅛ teaspoon (0.5ml) of vanilla absolute.

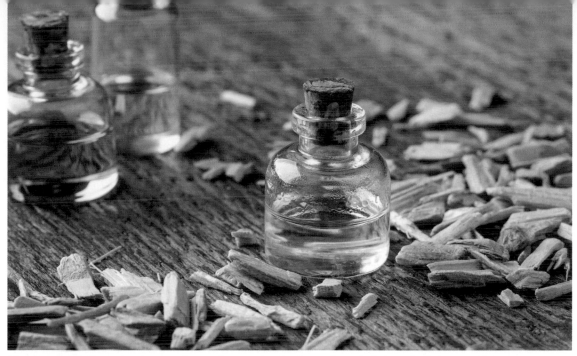
Wood essential oils are deeply grounding, and massaging the feet at the end of a long day helps to mitigate stress and anxiety.

FRANKINCENSE AND MYRRH FOOT MASSAGE OIL
MAKES 8 OUNCES (250ML)

Heal cracked skin and deeply soothe stressed muscles with this grounding oil full of skin-loving sesquiterpenes. Myrrh is a resin from the North African Commiphora tree, and myrrh resin has been used throughout history as a perfume, incense, and medicine. It has a light aroma that is deepened here by rich frankincense essential oil.

EQUIPMENT
- Glass bottle
- Funnel
- Glass measuring cup
- Measuring spoons

INGREDIENTS
Carrier Oils:
- 4 ounces (125ml) almond oil
- 3 ounces (90ml) olive oil
- 1 ounce (15ml) avocado oil

Essential Oils:
- 1 teaspoon (5ml) myrrh
- ½ teaspoon (2.5ml) frankincense

HOW TO MAKE
1. Add the carrier oils to a bottle with the funnel.
2. Add the essential oils.
3. Cap and gently swirl to incorporate.

HOW TO USE
Use this massage oil on your feet after a long day to promote relaxation and stress relief.

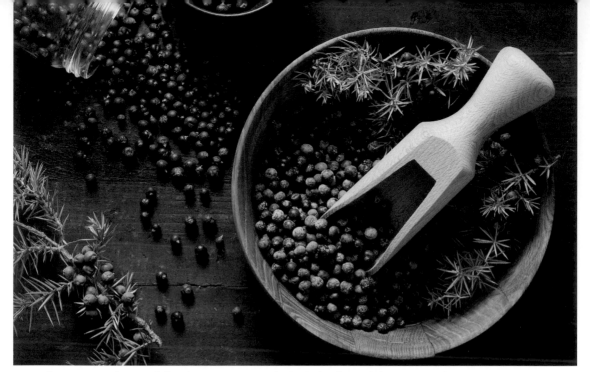

Juniper berries emit a fresh and slightly peppery essential oil, which is beautifully paired with bright bergamot.

JUNIPER BERRY BERGAMOT BACK RUB OIL
MAKES 8 OUNCES (250ML)

Refreshing bergamot is related to orange but is a bit spicier in its aromatic profile. It has a wonderful synergy with the fresh, peppery juniper berry and creates one of my very favorite blends. Enjoy an uplifting and stress-busting massage from someone you love enhanced by this highly aromatic and pleasure-inducing massage oil that is full of antioxidants like vitamin E to nurture your skin.

EQUIPMENT
- Glass bottle
- Funnel
- Glass measuring cup
- Measuring spoons

INGREDIENTS
Carrier Oils:
- 4 ounces (125ml) grapeseed, almond, or avocado oil
- 4 ounces (125ml) sunflower oil

Essential Oils:
- 1 teaspoon (5ml) bergamot
- ½ teaspoon (2.5ml) juniper berry

HOW TO MAKE
1. Add the carrier oils to a bottle with the funnel.
2. Add the essential oils.
3. Cap and gently swirl to incorporate.

HOW TO USE
Use this back massage oil for release and relaxation.

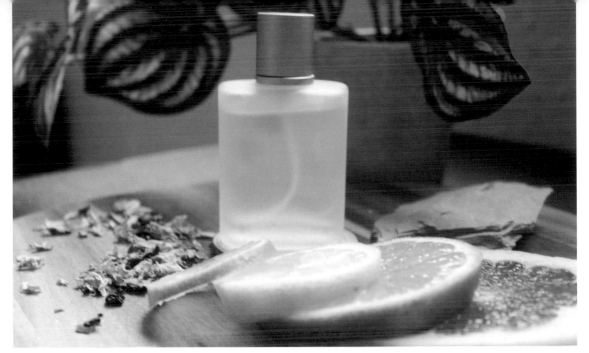

The secret to this blend is the ambrosial mix of fruits and flowers, delivering their uplifting chemical profiles directly to your brain.

BLISS MIST FRUIT AND FLOWER AMBROSIA SPRAY
MAKES ONE 2-OUNCE (60ML) BOTTLE

This light and ethereal, mood-lifting spray blends fruits and flowers to create a naturally refreshing boost. The grounding and serenity-producing rose and ylang ylang combine with the vibrant and enlivening trio of citrus finished off with the bright aroma of lemon myrtle. Carry in your bag or leave on your desk to restore a sense of balance and strengthen joy and optimism whenever you need it.

EQUIPMENT
- 2-ounce (60ml) spray bottle
- Measuring spoons
- Glass pipettes

INGREDIENTS
Base:
- 2 ounces (60ml) perfumer's alcohol

Essential Oils:
- ¼ teaspoon (1.25ml) + 8 drops pink grapefruit
- ⅛ teaspoon (0.5ml) tangerine
- 8 drops lemon
- 6 drops lemon myrtle
- 4 drops rose otto
- 2 drops ylang ylang

HOW TO MAKE
1. Add each essential oil to your spray bottle.
2. Fill the remainder with perfumer's alcohol and add the cap.

HOW TO USE
Leave in your bag or at your desk and spritz into your face, breathing deeply whenever you need a moment of pause to calm anxiety or lift your mood. Can also be used as a room, linen, or bathroom spray.

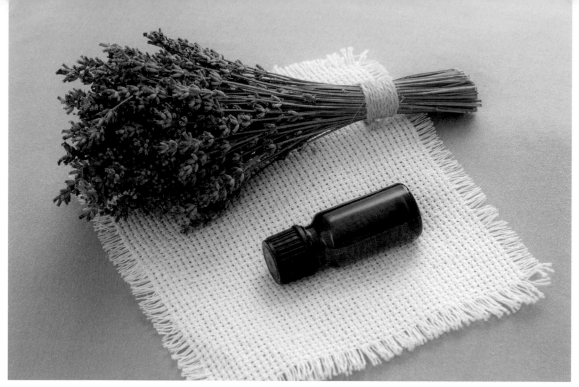

This mix makes a perfect gift for friends and family—we can all use a bit of relaxation at bedtime.

FLORAL FOREST BEDTIME PILLOW MIST
MAKES ONE 2-OUNCE (60ML) BOTTLE

Prepare yourself for deep, relaxing slumber with a few mists of this sedative, aromatic spray on your pillow and bed linens. Jasmine, rose, cedar, and lavender work synergistically to calm the nervous system and quiet the mind, for an uninterrupted and restorative night's sleep.

EQUIPMENT
- 2-ounce (60ml) spray bottle
- Measuring spoons
- Glass pipettes

INGREDIENTS
Base:
- 2 ounces (60ml) perfumer's alcohol

Essential Oils:
- ¼ teaspoon (1.25ml) lavender
- ¼ teaspoon (1.25ml) rose in jojoba
- ⅛ teaspoon (0.5ml) jasmine, optional
- 1 drop cedarwood

HOW TO MAKE
1. Add each essential oil to your spray bottle.
2. Fill the remainder with perfumer's alcohol and add the cap.

HOW TO USE
Spray your pillows, linens, and face before bedtime. Breathe deeply and slowly to induce a long, restorative night's sleep.

TIP: Swap the perfumer's alcohol for lavender hydrosol for an all-natural treat.

FRANKINCENSE ROSE CALMING SPRAY

MAKES ONE 2-OUNCE (60ML) BOTTLE

When life requires a respite, take a moment to breath in the gentle and comforting aroma of rose and frankincense. Rose is a true treasure of the essential oil world, requiring 60,000 roses to make a single ounce of precious essential oil. Frankincense has been used for thousands of years for its immunity-enhancing, antibacterial and antifungal qualities and is protective, purifying, and grounding. This blend is a natural way to support a balanced, tranquil mood.

EQUIPMENT
- 2-ounce (60ml) spray bottle
- Measuring spoons

INGREDIENTS
Base:
- 2 ounces (60ml) perfumer's alcohol

Essential Oils:
- 1 teaspoon (5ml) frankincense
- ¼ teaspoon (1.25ml) rose otto

HOW TO MAKE
1. Add each essential oil to your spray bottle.
2. Fill the remainder with perfumer's alcohol and add the cap.

HOW TO USE
Spritz into the face and breathe deeply and slowly anytime you need a respite from your surroundings.

BERGAMOT NEROLI TRAVEL ENDURANCE MIST

MAKES ONE 2-OUNCE (60ML) BOTTLE

Travel taxes our immune systems as well as our sense of calm and well-being—taking us out of our normal routines and putting us in crowded, hectic spaces that aren't always ideal. This mist blends neroli's powerful antidepressant and antitrauma properties with bergamot's stress-relieving and antiviral, antibacterial monoterpenes, and calming clary sage to make traveling far more pleasant. (**Full disclosure:** this blend smells WAY too good to only use for travel—I carry it in my purse all the time, as I'm addicted to the sweet and comforting aroma.)

EQUIPMENT
- 2-ounce (60ml) spray bottle
- Measuring spoons
- Glass pipettes

INGREDIENTS
Base:
- 2 ounces (60ml) perfumer's alcohol

Essential Oils:
- ¾ teaspoon (3.75ml) bergamot
- 8 drops neroli
- 3 drops clary sage

HOW TO MAKE
1. Add each essential oil to your spray bottle.
2. Fill the remainder with perfumer's alcohol and add the cap.

HOW TO USE
Spritz into the face and breathe deeply and slowly anytime you need a respite and protection from the assault of your surroundings, whether on a train, plane, subway, or other hectic, crowded space.

Making your own cleansers and home products is one of the easiest changes you can make to improve your life and health.

HOME CARE RECIPES

One of the most insidious ways we're exposed to chemicals happens inside our most intimate of spaces: our homes. From the off-gassing of new furniture and appliances to all the commercial cleansers, detergents, and sprays, we can unwittingly create harmful spaces. You can avoid these chemicals is by making your own cleaning and home products from just a few safe, natural ingredients.

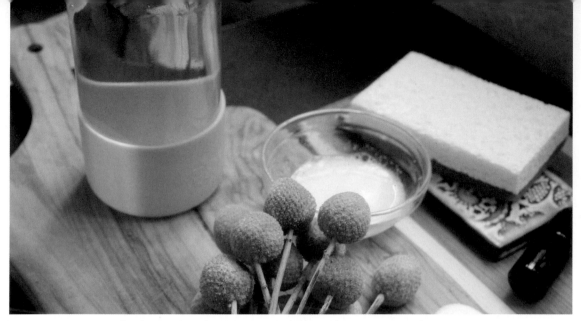

Lemon verbena essential oil has antifungal and antimicrobial chemical constituents, making it a natural for kitchen cleanup.

LEMON VERBENA KITCHEN CLEANSER
MAKES 16 OUNCES (500ML)

While the disinfectant properties of the soap ingredients go to work, the vibrant and fresh scent of lemon verbena offers pure pleasure, taking the tedium out of cleaning with its mood-lifting and stress-busting chemistry.

EQUIPMENT

- Large glass measuring cup
- 16-ounce (500ml) glass spray bottle
- Funnel
- Measuring cup
- Measuring spoons
- Wooden stir stick or stirring spoon

INGREDIENTS

Base:

- 2 cups (500ml) distilled water
- 1 teaspoon (5ml) borax
- 1 teaspoon (5ml) liquid castile soap
- ½ teaspoon (2.5ml) washing soda

Essential Oil:

- 1 tablespoon (15ml) lemon verbena

HOW TO MAKE

1. Pour the distilled water into the measuring cup and heat it in the microwave for about 1 minute, or until warm to the touch.
2. Add the remaining ingredients and stir.
3. Pour through the funnel into the spray bottle.

HOW TO USE

Use to clean your sink, countertops, and any surfaces that require cleaning.

TIP: For a luxurious variation, substitute the distilled water with lemon, orange, or neroli hydrosol and skip the essential oil.

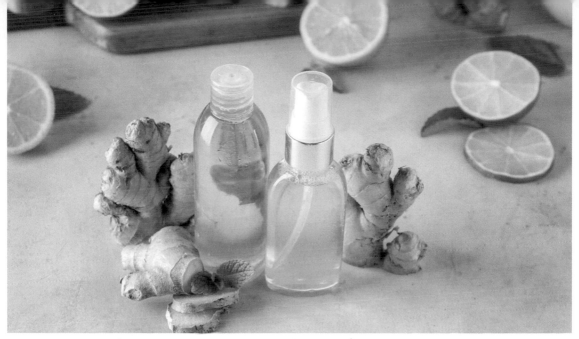

This disinfectant deep cleans while smelling like an energizing, tropical escape!

GINGER LIME DISINFECTANT SPRAY
MAKES 16 OUNCES (500ML)

Keep this spray on hand wherever you want quick access to light cleaning touch-ups, deep cleaning, or spot treatments. Ginger and lime essential oils make a natural aromatic pairing, and both offer strong antibacterial qualities.

EQUIPMENT
- 16-ounce (500ml) glass spray bottle
- Funnel
- Pipette
- Measuring cups
- Measuring spoons

INGREDIENTS
Base:
- 1 cup (250ml) water
- 1 cup (250ml) white vinegar
- 2 tablespoons (30ml) rubbing alcohol

Essential Oils:
- ½ teaspoon (2.5ml) lime
- 8 drops ginger

HOW TO MAKE
1. Pour the water and vinegar through the funnel into the spray bottle. Add the rubbing alcohol.
2. Drop in the essential oils and put on the top. Shake to mix.

HOW TO USE
Essential oils will not permanently disperse into water or alcohol, so shake before each use. Spray onto countertops, sinks, or anywhere that needs cleaning.

TIP: For a luxurious variation, substitute the water with lime or yuzu hydrosol.

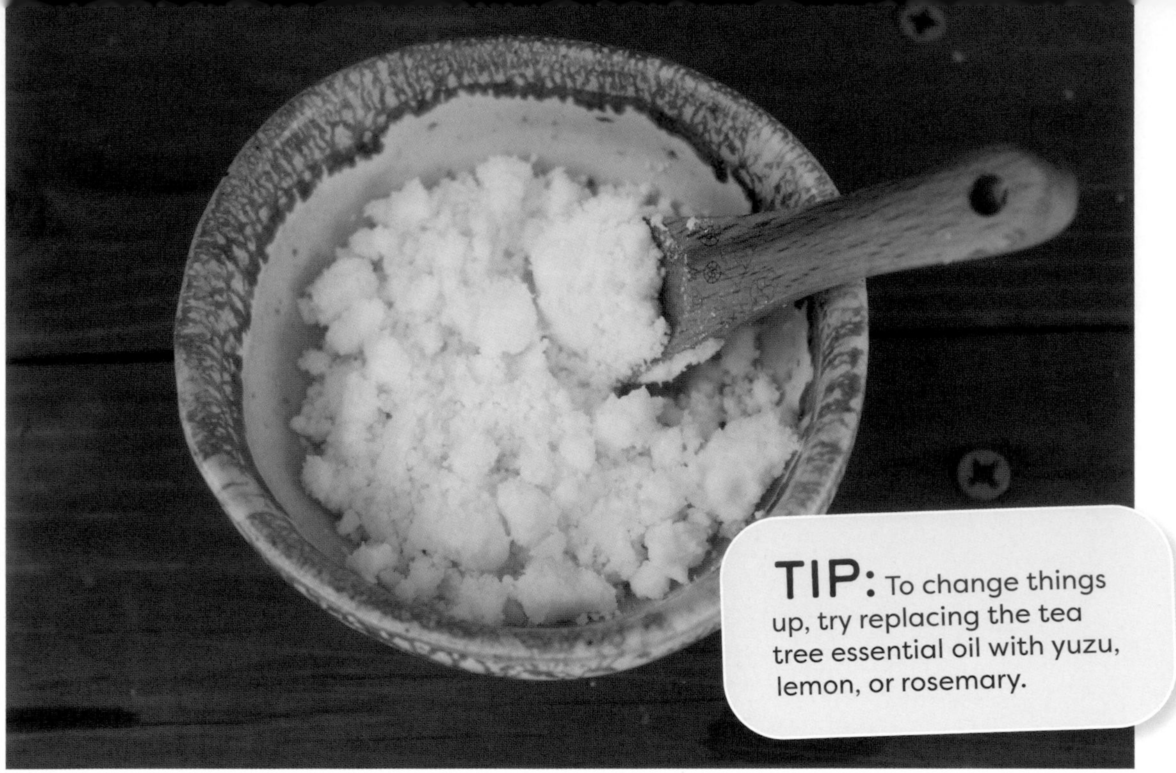

This scrub works naturally works wonders without harsh chemicals or waste.

TEA TREE TOILET SCRUB

MAKES 8 OUNCES (250ML)

This scrubby little cleanser keeps your toilet area clean and disinfected, naturally.

EQUIPMENT

- 8-ounce (250ml) glass or ceramic jar
- Mixing bowl
- Stirring spoon
- Measuring spoons
- Pipette

INGREDIENTS

Base:

- ¾ cup (175ml) baking soda
- ¼ cup (60ml) castile soap
- 1 tablespoon (15ml) fine salt
- 1 tablespoon (15ml) water

Essential Oil:

- 12 drops tea tree

HOW TO MAKE

1. Add all the ingredients to the mixing bowl and stir. Press with the back of the spoon to smooth out clumps and fully incorporate all the ingredients.
2. Transfer to the jar and cap.

HOW TO USE

Place around 1 tablespoon (15ml) into the toilet bowl or onto your scrub brush. Clean the bowl as normal, flushing to rinse.

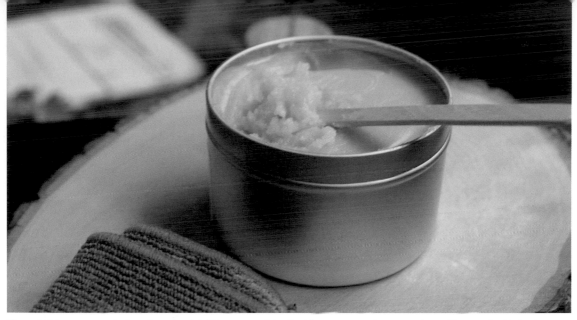

The polishing powers of plant-based candelilla wax combined with orange wax is a natural emollient and adds to the wonderful aroma of this wood polishing wax.

ORANGE WOOD SHINE WAX

MAKES 8 OUNCES (250ML)

We've left the bees alone with this flower-wax wood polish, enhanced with orange wax, a derivative of orange peels that has a highly concentrated orange scent. With a towel and just a bit of elbow grease, your wood surfaces will shimmer and shine.

EQUIPMENT

- 8-ounce (250ml) tin or glass jar
- Glass measuring cup
- Additional measuring cup
- Measuring spoons
- Wooden stir stick

INGREDIENTS

Base:

- ¾ cup (175ml) olive oil, almond oil, or avocado oil
- ¼ cup (30g) candelilla wax
- 1 tablespoon (15ml) orange wax

Essential Oil:

- ¼ teaspoon (1.25ml) sweet orange

HOW TO MAKE

1. Fill the measuring cup with the oil and add the candelilla wax.
2. Microwave for 1 minute and then stop to stir. Return to the microwave and heat in 30-second increments, stopping to stir in between. Stop before the mixture is fully melted to avoid overheating. Stir until completely melted.
3. Add the orange wax and essential oil. Stir to incorporate.
4. Pour into the container and allow to sit uncovered for 2 hours.
5. Once fully solidified, cap. Your wax is now ready to use!

HOW TO USE

Place about 1 tablespoon (15ml) onto a dry cloth or directly onto the wood surface. Massage into the wood with a circular motion. Let the wax absorb into the wood; don't wash it off. The oils and wax will create a protective barrier and leave the wood looking (and smelling) great.

This powder leaves your carpets with a light, soft texture and a beautiful scent.

GERANIUM CARPET POWDER

MAKES 16 OUNCES (500ML)

Freshen up rugs and carpets with this easy carpet powder made with ingredients you probably have on hand. The geranium essential oil is antimicrobial and antibacterial, with a vibrant, herbaceous scent that calms the nerves.

EQUIPMENT

- Shaker tube or can
- Mixing bowl
- Stirring spoon
- Measuring spoons

INGREDIENTS

Base:
- 1 cup (250ml) baking soda
- ½ cup (125ml) cornstarch or arrowroot powder
- ½ cup (125ml) Epsom salt

Essential Oil:
- 2 teaspoons (10ml) geranium

HOW TO MAKE

1. Add the base ingredients to the mixing bowl. Stir to incorporate.
2. Add the essential oil and stir to mix.
3. Transfer to the container and cap.

HOW TO USE

Sprinkle over your carpet, either allowing it to sit before vacuuming or vacuuming immediately. (Use conservatively on darker carpets.)

LEMON MYRTLE DISHWASHING POWDER

MAKES 32 OUNCES (1L)

Keep chemicals off your kitchenware with this natural dishwasher detergent powered by vibrant and antibacterial lemon myrtle essential oil.

EQUIPMENT

- 32-ounce (1L) jar, tin, bucket, or burlap bag
- Measuring cup
- Measuring spoons
- Mixing bowl
- Wooden stir stick or stirring spoon

INGREDIENTS

Base:
- 1 cup (250ml) borax
- 1 cup (250ml) washing soda
- 1 cup (250ml) baking soda
- ½ cup (125ml) citric acid
- ½ cup (125ml) salt

Essential Oil:
- 1 teaspoon (5ml) lemon myrtle

HOW TO MAKE

1. Add the base ingredients to the mixing bowl and stir to incorporate, pressing out clumps.
2. Add the essential oil, press out clumps with the back of the spoon, then stir to incorporate.
3. Transfer to chosen container.

HOW TO USE

Add 1 tablespoon (15ml) to your dishwasher's detergent compartment for each load. For a rinsing agent, use white vinegar.

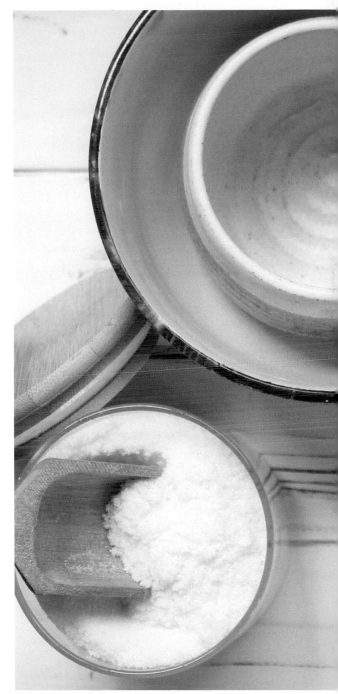

Bypass the plastic-covered pods by making your own natural and effective dishwasher detergent with just a few simple ingredients.

MANDARIN THYME GLASS CLEANER
MAKES 16 OUNCES (500ML)

Clear your mind and your windows: vinegar and water make an excellent natural glass cleaner, with red mandarin and thyme offering antifungal properties and the joy of an uplifting crisp and clean scent.

EQUIPMENT
- 16-ounce (500ml) glass spray bottle
- Glass measuring cup
- Measuring spoons
- Funnel

INGREDIENTS
Base:
- 1 cup (250ml) white vinegar
- 1 cup (250ml) water

Essential Oil:
- ½ teaspoon (2.5ml) red mandarin
- 4–6 drops thyme

HOW TO MAKE
1. Add all the ingredients to the bottle through the funnel.
2. Add the spritz top and swirl to mix.

HOW TO USE
Spray onto glass before wiping with newspaper, a microfiber cloth, or a paper towel.

PINE MANDARIN WOOD CLEANSER
MAKES 16 OUNCES (500ML)

Clean and restore the wood surfaces in your home naturally with this vinegar- and oil-based cleanser featuring pine needle essential oil. True pine essential oil is nothing like the artificial scent found in many commercial cleansers: its fresh, clean, and woody aroma is transportive and its antifungal properties are a bonus.

EQUIPMENT
- 16-ounce (500ml) glass spray bottle
- Glass measuring cup
- Measuring spoons
- Funnel

INGREDIENTS
Base:
- 1 cup (250ml) white vinegar
- 1 cup (250ml) olive oil or fractionated coconut oil
- 1 tablespoon (15ml) liquid castile soap

Essential Oils:
- 1 tablespoon (15ml) red, yellow, or green mandarin
- 2 teaspoons (10ml) pine

HOW TO MAKE
1. Pour all the ingredients through the funnel into the spray bottle.
2. Add the mister top and shake gently to blend.

HOW TO USE
Spray onto any wood that needs cleaning, then wipe to dry. Double the recipe to add to a bucket for mopping floors.

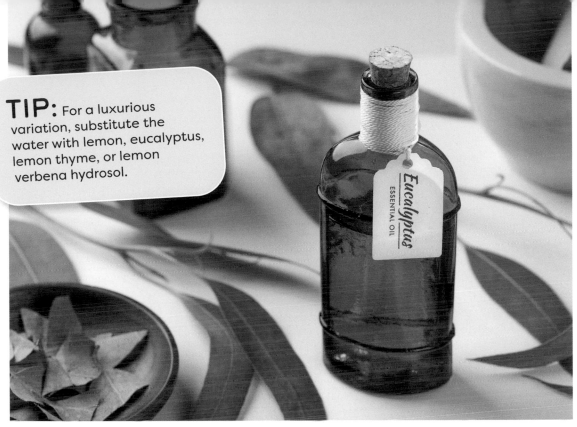

TIP: For a luxurious variation, substitute the water with lemon, eucalyptus, lemon thyme, or lemon verbena hydrosol.

This clothing rinse is perfect for clothes that aren't safe for machine washing.

EUCALYPTUS CLOTHING RINSE
MAKES 16 OUNCES (500ML)

For delicate clothes we don't want tumbling at high heats, use this natural rinse instead. It's gentle and leaves your valuables clean and supremely cared for, ready to lay out to dry. *Makes a single use.*

EQUIPMENT
- 16-ounce (500ml) jar, bottle, or jug
- Measuring cup
- Measuring spoons
- Stirring spoon

INGREDIENTS
Base:
- 2 cups (500ml) water
- ½ cup (125ml) baking soda

Essential Oils:
- ⅛ teaspoon (0.5ml) eucalyptus

HOW TO MAKE
1. Add all ingredients to the jar or bottle.
2. Stir to combine.

HOW TO USE
Fill a small tub with warm water and add all of the clothing rinse. Swish to mix. Add your clothes and let them soak for 5 to 10 minutes before rinsing and hanging to dry.

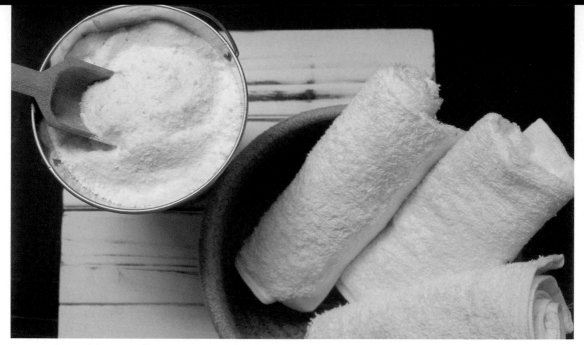

A scoop or two of this natural laundry detergent leaves your clothes fluffy and clean, without the buildup created from soap-based detergents.

BERGAMOT LAUNDRY SOAP
MAKES 4 CUPS (1L)

This recipe is easy, soap-free, and does the job with the power of natural ingredients and essential oils. It also doesn't leave a buildup on your clothes, so you'll find them fresh and fluffy.

EQUIPMENT

- 32-ounce (1L) repurposed carton, pail, jar, or bucket
- Measuring cups
- Measuring spoons
- Mixing bowl
- Stirring spoon

INGREDIENTS

Base:

- 2 cups (500ml) washing soda
- 2 cups (500ml) baking soda
- ⅔ cup (150ml) Epsom salt
- 3 tablespoons (45ml) fine sea salt (white, pink, or a mixture)

Essential Oil:

- 1 teaspoon (5ml) bergamot

HOW TO MAKE

1. Add all the ingredients to the mixing bowl, essential oil last, and stir to mix.
2. Using the back of the spoon, spend some time pressing out all the clumps to make one uniform consistency.
3. Transfer to the container and cap.

HOW TO USE

Add ¼ cup (60ml) to a medium load of laundry, adjusting for the size of load as needed.

TIP: Customize your laundry soap by replacing the bergamot essential oil with any oil you love. Rosemary, lemon, and lavender all work well.

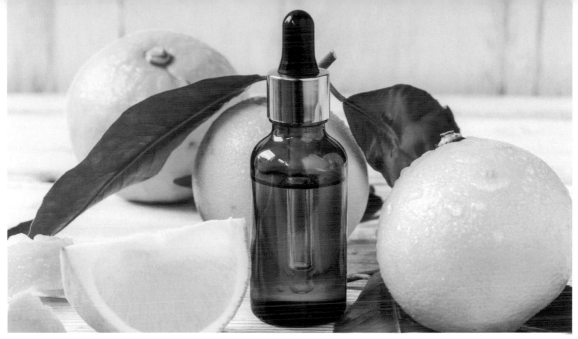

This stain remover combines powerful natural cleaning agents with stimulating lemon and eucalyptus essential oils.

LEMON STAIN REMOVER
MAKES 2 OUNCES (60ML)

Catching a stain early with this natural remover will restore your item and make it as good as new. Keep a bottle handy for all such small emergencies.

EQUIPMENT
- Glass measuring cup
- Measuring spoons
- Pipettes
- Wooden stir stick
- Funnel
- 2-ounce (60ml) glass dropper bottle

INGREDIENTS
Base:
- ¼ cup (60ml) white vinegar
- ½ tablespoon (7ml) baking soda
- 1 teaspoon (5ml) fine salt
- 1 teaspoon (5ml) water

Essential Oils:
- 12 drops lemon
- 4 drops eucalyptus

HOW TO MAKE
1. Add the vinegar, salt, and baking soda to the glass measuring cup. (The baking soda will cause it to foam up, so be sure you're working in a larger container before pouring it into the bottle.)
2. Add the essential oils and water, and stir.
3. Pour through the funnel into the dropper bottle.

HOW TO USE
Apply a few drops to the stain and let sit anywhere from a few minutes to a couple hours before washing.

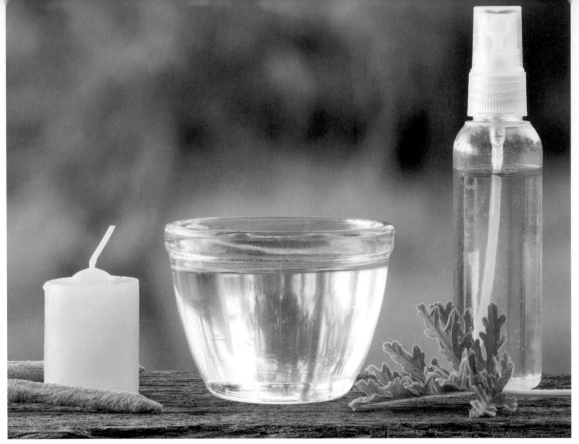

This is a must-make recipe for keeping summertime fun sting- and bite-free.

BUG REPELLANT SPRAY
MAKES 1 OUNCE (30 ML)

For an as-needed weapon against critter assaults, keep this spray on hand. Mist onto exposed skin, clothing, picnic tablecloths, and other surfaces to deter creepy crawlers and bug bites.

EQUIPMENT
- 1-ounce (30ml) spray bottle
- Measuring spoons
- Funnel

INGREDIENTS
Base:
- 1 ounce (30ml) perfumer's alcohol, witch hazel, or isopropyl alcohol

Essential Oil:
- ¼ teaspoon (1.25ml) citronella

HOW TO MAKE
1. Add the perfumer's alcohol to the bottle through the funnel.
2. Add the essential oil.
3. Cap and shake to blend.

HOW TO USE
Mist onto your clothes and any exposed skin to naturally repel mosquitos.

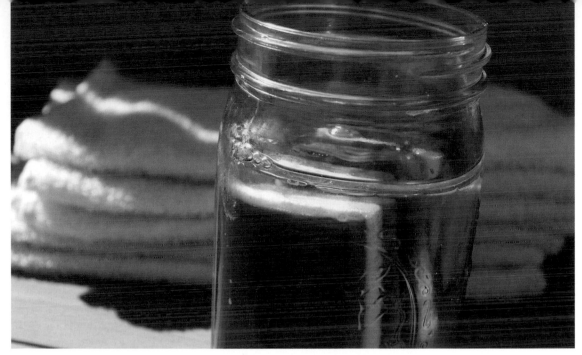

The thickness of your fabric will determine how many sheets you can make at one time.

ESSENTIAL OIL DRYER SHEETS
MAKES AT LEAST 12 DRYER SHEETS

It's easy to make reusable dryer sheets with this recipe that repurposes old cloth and fabric scraps.

EQUIPMENT
- 16-ounce (500ml) wide-mouth glass jar
- 6" x 6" (15.2 x 15.2cm) fabric squares, reusable cloth baby wipes, or baby wash cloths

INGREDIENTS
Base:
- 1 cup (250ml) white vinegar or cleaning vinegar

Essential Oil:
- 2 teaspoons (10ml) oil of choice (I recommend lavender, pine, tangerine, rosemary, geranium, peppermint, or eucalyptus. You can use single scents or blends like lavender and eucalyptus, orange and peppermint, or pine and rosemary.)

HOW TO MAKE
1. Add the ingredients to the glass jar. Shake to blend.
2. Fold the cloth pieces and place them in the jar. Cap the jar and turn it upside down to distribute the liquid into the cloth, then turn right side up.

HOW TO USE
After placing your clothes in the dryer, take a piece of cloth from the prepared jar and place it in the dryer—the vinegar scent will burn off, leaving the essential oil aromas behind.

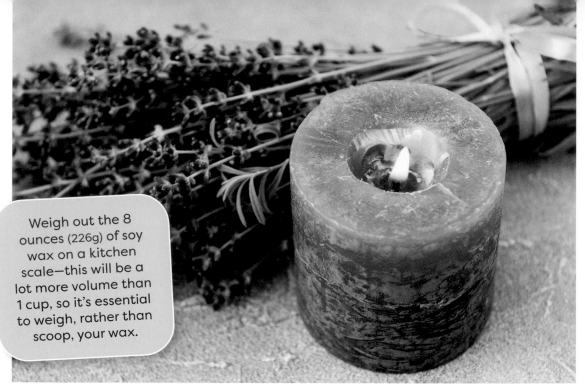

Weigh out the 8 ounces (226g) of soy wax on a kitchen scale—this will be a lot more volume than 1 cup, so it's essential to weigh, rather than scoop, your wax.

Candles offer unliminited opportunities for creativity—explore different colorants, botanicals, and other decorative elements to make them all your own.

ROSEMARY LAVENDER CANDLE
MAKES ONE 8-OUNCE (226G) CANDLE

Candles are easier than you might think to make, and you can save significant cash making your own if you burn candles often. Once you purchase the basic ingredient—soy wax—plus the wicks and containers, you're good to go any time the desire for fire strikes. These two-ingredient candles offer the healthiest way to burn and breathe, without the toxic chemicals you'll find in many commercial candles.

EQUIPMENT
- Double boiler
- 8-ounce (250ml) candle holder
- Wicks with adhesive
- Glass measuring cup
- Measuring spoons
- Kitchen scale
- 4 wooden craft sticks or clothespins

INGREDIENTS
Base:
- 8 ounces (226g) soy wax flakes
- ½ teaspoon (2.5ml) lavender mica or purple crayon for color, optional
- Sprinkling of lavender petals, rosemary leaves, or both, optional

Essential Oils:
- 1 teaspoon (5ml) lavender
- ½ teaspoon (2.5ml) rosemary

HOW TO MAKE

1. Melt the soy wax in the double boiler over low heat, stirring occasionally, until fully melted. Add the colorant, if using.
2. While the wax is melting, prepare your candle holder by attaching the wick to the bottom with the double-sided adhesive squares.
3. Remove the wax from the heat and add the essential oils. Stir.
4. Pour into the candle holder and sprinkle with the lavender petals or rosemary leaves, if using.
5. Place a wooden craft stick or clothespin horizontally across the top of the candle holder on either side of the wick to hold it up straight in the center of the candle and keep it from falling to the side.
6. Wipe any leftover wax out of the double boiler pot with a paper towel before it hardens and throw out any used stir sticks.
7. Allow the candle to set for 2 to 4 hours before cutting the wick to the desired length (I cut mine just above the top of the holder). Your candle is ready to use!

HOW TO USE

Light the wick and enjoy the fresh, invigorating fragrance.

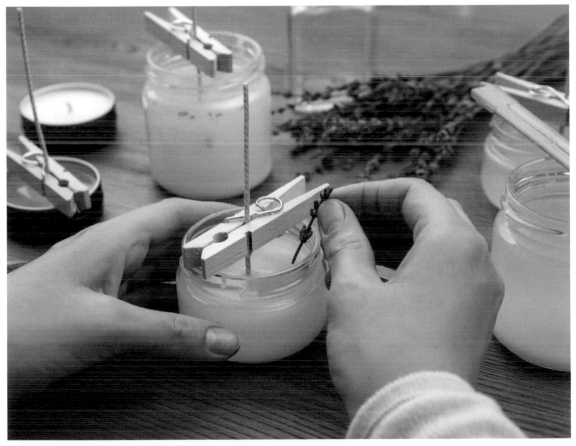

You need to keep the wicks straight while the candle wax hardens. Use wooden clothespins or place wooden craft sticks on either side of the wick.

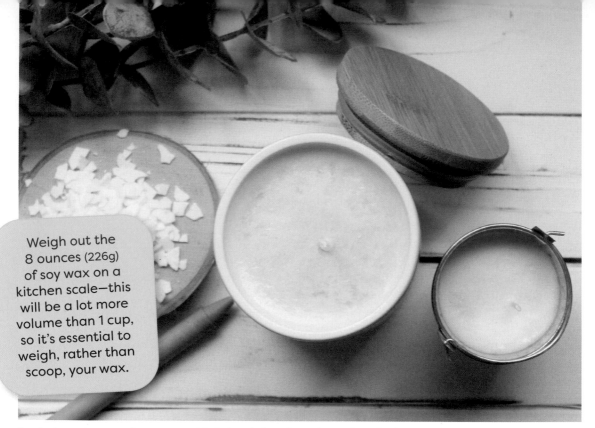

Weigh out the 8 ounces (226g) of soy wax on a kitchen scale—this will be a lot more volume than 1 cup, so it's essential to weigh, rather than scoop, your wax.

Eucalyptus and peppermint are accessible, beloved oils and together pack a refreshing punch.

EUCALYPTUS MINT CANDLE

MAKES ONE 8-OUNCE (226G) CANDLE

When your space needs clearing and freshening with an energy uplift, let eucalyptus and peppermint go to work via this natural soy-based candle.

EQUIPMENT

- Double boiler
- 8-ounce (250ml) candle holder
- Wicks with adhesive
- Glass measuring cup
- Measuring spoons
- Kitchen scale
- 4 wooden craft sticks or clothepins

INGREDIENTS

Base:

- 8 ounces (226g) soy wax flakes
- ½ teaspoon (2.5ml) green mica, spirulina, or crayon for color, optional (I used ½ of a large green crayon for my candle)

Essential Oils:

- ¾ teaspoon (3.75ml) eucalyptus
- ¾ teaspoon (3.75ml) peppermint

HOW TO MAKE

1. Melt the soy wax in the double boiler over low heat, stirring occasionally, until fully melted. Add the colorant, if using.
2. While the wax is melting, prepare your candle holder by attaching the wick to the bottom with the double-sided adhesive squares.
3. Remove the wax from the heat and add the essential oils. Stir.
4. Pour into the candle holder.
5. Place a wooden craft stick or clothespin horizontally across the top of the candle holder on either side of the wick to hold it up straight in the center of the candle and keep it from falling to the side.
6. Wipe any leftover wax out of the double boiler pot with a paper towel before it hardens and throw out any used stir sticks.
7. Allow the candle to set for 2 to 4 hours before cutting the wick to the desired length (I cut mine just above the top of the holder). Your candle is ready to use!

HOW TO USE

Light the wick and enjoy the fresh, invigorating fragrance.

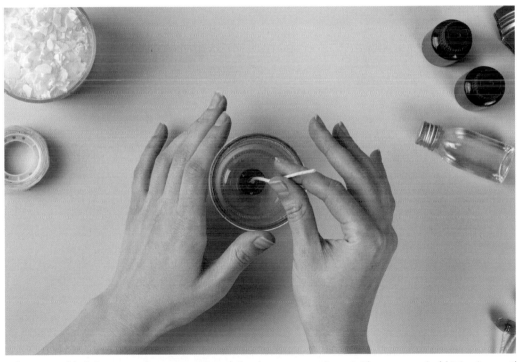

Adhesives will help keep you place your wick exactly where you want it to sit. Then you can hold it in place as the candle dries using wooden craft sticks or a clothespin.

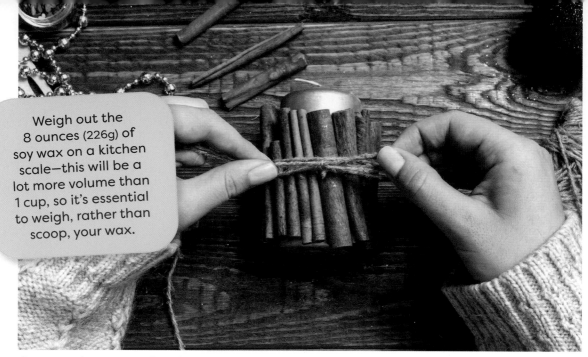

> Weigh out the 8 ounces (226g) of soy wax on a kitchen scale—this will be a lot more volume than 1 cup, so it's essential to weigh, rather than scoop, your wax.

The aromas of cinnamon and vanilla add warm comfort to any space.

CINNAMON VANILLA CANDLE
MAKES ONE 8-OUNCE (226G) CANDLE

Add a bit of spice and the grounding affects of vanilla to your space with this seductive and warming candle.

EQUIPMENT
- Double boiler
- 8-ounce (250ml) candle holder
- Wicks with adhesive
- Glass measuring cup
- Measuring spoons
- Kitchen scale
- 4 wooden craft sticks or clothespins

INGREDIENTS
Base:
- 8 ounces (226g) soy wax flakes
- Cinnamon powder or gold mica for color, optional
- Cinnamon sticks, dried vanilla beans, raffia ribbon, or twine for decoration, optional

Essential Oils:
- 1 teaspoon (5ml) vanilla absolute
- 2 drops cinnamon

HOW TO MAKE

1. Melt the soy wax in the double boiler over low heat, stirring occasionally, until fully melted. Add the cinnamon powder or gold mica, if using. Stir and adjust the cinnamon or gold mica until the desired color is reached.

2. While the wax is melting, prepare your candle holder by attaching the wick to the bottom with the double-sided adhesive squares.

3. Remove the wax from the heat and add the essential oils. Stir.

4. Pour into the candle holder.

5. Place a wooden craft stick or clothespin horizontally across the top of the candle holder on either side of the wick to hold it up straight in the center of the candle and keep it from falling to the side.

6. Wipe any leftover wax out of the double boiler pot with a paper towel before it hardens and throw out any used stir sticks.

7. Allow the candle to set for 2 to 4 hours before cutting the wick to the desired length (I cut mine just above the top of the holder). Top with a dried vanilla bean or cinnamon stick, if using, for decoration. Your candle is ready to use!

HOW TO USE

Light the wick and enjoy the fresh, invigorating fragrance.

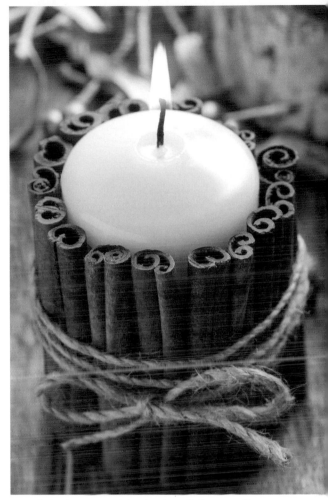

Use whole cinnamon sticks, dried vanilla beans, raffia ribbons, or twine to add a rustic cheerfulness to your finished candles.

JASMINE ORANGE CANDLE

MAKES ONE 8-OUNCE (226G) CANDLE

The sultry and seductive aromas of sweet orange and jasmine create an ambience of luxury and sublime sensuality.

EQUIPMENT
- Double boiler
- 8-ounce (250ml) candle holder
- Wicks with adhesive
- Glass measuring cup
- Measuring spoons
- Kitchen scale
- 4 wooden craft sticks or clothespins

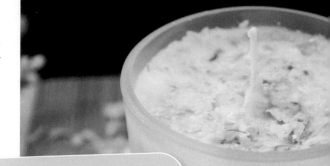

Weigh out the 8 ounces (226g) of soy wax on a kitchen scale—this will be a lot more volume than 1 cup, so it's essential to weigh, rather than scoop, your wax.

INGREDIENTS

Base:
- 8 ounces (226g) soy wax flakes
- ½ teaspoon (2.5ml) orange mica, turmeric, orange clay, or crayon for color, optional
- Sprinkling of dried jasmine petals, optional

Essential Oils:
- 2 teaspoons (10ml) sweet orange
- ½ teaspoon (2.5ml) jasmine

HOW TO MAKE

1. Melt the soy wax in the double boiler over low heat, stirring occasionally, until fully melted. Add the colorant, if using.
2. While the wax is melting, prepare your candle holder by attaching the wick to the bottom with the double-sided adhesive squares.
3. Remove the wax from the heat and add the essential oils. Stir.
4. Pour into the candle holder and sprinkle with the dried jasmine petals, if using.
5. Place a wooden craft stick or clothespin horizontally across the top of the candle holder on either side of the wick to hold it up straight in the center in the candle and keep it from falling to the side.

Personalize your candles with natural colorants and dried fruits and flowers for a unique creation.

6. Wipe any leftover wax out of the double boiler pot with a paper towel before it hardens and throw out any used stir sticks.
7. Allow the candle to set for 2 to 4 hours before cutting the wick to the desired length (I cut mine just above the top of the holder. Your candle is ready to use!

HOW TO USE
Light the wick and enjoy the fresh, invigorating fragrance.

SENSUAL ROOM SPRAY

MAKES ONE 2-OUNCE (60ML)
SPRAY BOTTLE

This luxurious spray creates a heady, sensual ambiance, with the sweetness of jasmine and vanilla balanced by the freshness of neroli flower. So good you'll want to wear it as perfume (and you're more than welcome to)!

EQUIPMENT
- 2-ounce (60ml) spray bottle
- Pipettes
- Funnel

INGREDIENTS
Base:
- 2 ounces (60ml) perfumer's alcohol

Essential Oils:
- 3 drops vanilla absolute
- 20 drops jasmine
- 5 drops neroli

HOW TO MAKE
1. Use a clean pipette to add each essential oil to the spray bottle.
2. Fill the remainder with perfumer's alcohol through the funnel. Cap the bottle.

HOW TO USE
Spray throughout your house to naturally freshen up any rooms that need it or to create a certain aromatic ambiance.

UPLIFTING ROOM SPRAY

MAKES ONE 2-OUNCE (60ML)
SPRAY BOTTLE

When you want to create an upbeat mood with positive vibrations, you can't go wrong with this fresh and lively citrus trio.

EQUIPMENT
- 2-ounce (60ml) spray bottle
- Pipettes
- Funnel

INGREDIENTS
Base:
- 2 ounces (60ml) perfumer's alcohol

Essential Oils:
- 16 drops pink grapefruit
- 12 drops tangerine
- 6 drops bergamot

HOW TO MAKE
1. Use a clean pipette to add each essential oil to the spray bottle.
2. Fill the remainder with perfumer's alcohol through the funnel. Cap the bottle.

HOW TO USE
Spray throughout your house to naturally freshen up any rooms that need it or to create a certain aromatic ambiance.

TRANQUILITY ROOM SPRAY

MAKES ONE 2-OUNCE (60ML) SPRAY BOTTLE

What could be more relaxing than lounging in a field of flowers on a warm summer's day? Enjoy the next-best option whenever you want to slow time down and breathe just a little easier.

EQUIPMENT
- 2-ounce (60ml) spray bottle
- Pipettes
- Funnel

INGREDIENTS
Base:
- 2 ounces (60ml) perfumer's alcohol

Essential Oils:
- 22 drops rose in jojoba
- 8 drops lavender
- 1 drop chamomile

HOW TO MAKE
1. Use a clean pipette to add each essential oil to the spray bottle.
2. Fill the remainder with perfumer's alcohol through the funnel. Cap the bottle.

HOW TO USE
Mist rooms and your entranceway anytime, or before guests come over to create a peaceful, welcoming ambiance.

GROUNDING ROOM SPRAY

MAKES ONE 2-OUNCE (60ML) SPRAY BOTTLE

Bring your energy to a peaceful place with this trio of grounding scents that play wonderfully together: a wood scent, a root scent, and a grass scent for those days you just need to bring things down a notch.

EQUIPMENT
- 2-ounce (60ml) spray bottle
- Pipettes
- Funnel

INGREDIENTS
Base:
- 2 ounces (60ml) perfumer's alcohol

Essential Oils:
- 16 drops cedar
- 16 drops lemongrass
- 5 drops vetiver

HOW TO MAKE
1. Use a clean pipette to add each essential oil to the spray bottle.
2. Fill the remainder with perfumer's alcohol through the funnel. Cap the bottle.

HOW TO USE
Spray throughout your house to naturally freshen up any rooms that need it or to create a certain aromatic ambiance.

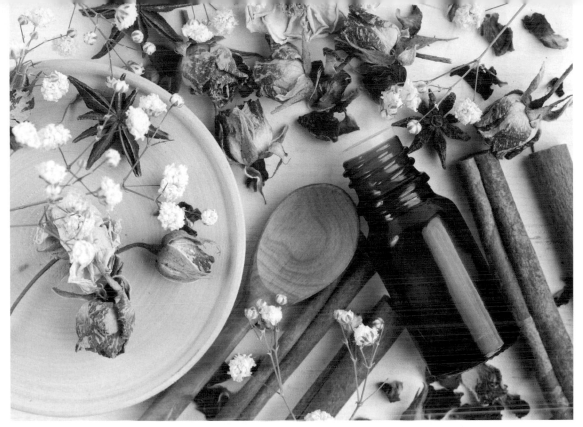

This spray has a warm scent that feels like soothing embrace.

COMFORT ROOM SPRAY
MAKES ONE 2-OUNCE (60ML) SPRAY BOTTLE

Homey and inspired by the coziness of the holidays, this citrus and spice blend induces feelings of safety and love, while making your home smell good enough to eat.

EQUIPMENT
- 2-ounce (60ml) spray bottle
- Pipettes
- Funnel

INGREDIENTS
Base:
- 2 ounces (60ml) perfumer's alcohol

Essential Oils:
- ¼ teaspoon (1.25ml) orange
- 1 drop cinnamon
- 1 drop clove

HOW TO MAKE
1. Use a clean pipette to add each essential oil to the spray bottle.
2. Fill the remainder with perfumer's alcohol through the funnel. Cap the bottle.

HOW TO USE
Spray throughout your house to naturally freshen up any rooms that need it or to create a certain aromatic ambiance.

About the Author

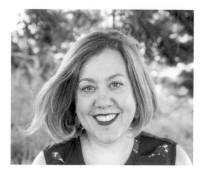

Stephanie Ariel is a certified aromatherapist, yoga teacher, and entrepreneur living in an adobe bungalow in the historic district of Santa Fe, New Mexico, with her dog Rexi. When she's not hiking the hills, swimming, or making natural products, she can be found running her online essential oils store, www.ArtisanAromatics.com.

Index

PHOTO CREDITS

Unless otherwise noted, all photography by Stephanie Ariel.

The following images are from Shutterstock.com: Front cover main image: ju_see; Front cover top right, 22–23, 28 jojoba, 30, 44, 91, 136, 168 bottom, 195: New Africa; 1: EKramar; 8, 25 butters: Africa Studio; 9: Ekaterina Glazkova; 14 peppermint: Egor Rodynchenko; 14 rose otto: Miglena Pencheva; 14 lavender: Soho A Studio; 14 frankincense, 15 vetiver: AmyLv; 15 cypress: Marinodenisenko; 15 tea tree: Gummy Bear; 15 sweet orange, 24 baking soda: Anton Starikov; 15 lemongrass: Wealthylady; 15 ylang ylang: NOPPHARAT9889; 24 aloe vera: Photoongraphy; 24 Borax: sulit.photos; 25 wax: Chadchai Krisadapong; 25 oils: AlenKadr; 26 citric acid: Ekaterina43; 26 colorants: Rostovtsevayu; 26 Dead Sea mud: Eirene Fagus; 26 exfoliants: beats1; 27 wax, 29 stearic acid: Meowcyber; 27 glycerin: Rassamee Design; 27 GSE: Liudmyla Guniavaia; 28 bottle: Shablon; 29 alcohol: Thammasak Lek; 29 pumice: ANATOL; 29 wax: Nataliia Trytenichenko; 31: kazmulka; 32–33: Pressmaster; 34 blender: Iryna Budanova; 34 double boiler: Arina P Habich; 34: electric mixer: BearFotos; 34 funnel: chanin1991; 35 scale: gresei; 35 measuring spoons: Hurst Photo; 35 bowls: Michal Dzierzynski; 35 mortar and pestle: bonchan; 35 pipette: Olha Kozachenko; 36 top: MT-R; 36 bottom: Atroshchenko Andrey; 37 thermometer: Susan Edmondson; 37 wax paper: this_baker; 37 wicks: MerlinTmb; 37 craft sticks: Sarah2; 37 stir sticks: Voravuth Chuanyou; 38 bottles: AKaiser; 38 glass jar: reinhardfenzl.com; 39 labels: Noppanun K; 39 label maker: rizalfaridz71; 39 paper tubes: Andriana Syvanych; 39 bottle: BOOCYS; 40 jars: Darknesssss; 40 shaker: Sonia Dubois; 40 bottles: Alina Yudina; 40 tins: DJ Srki; 45: UfaBizPhoto; 52: 5PH; 53: Tatevosian Yana; 63: Olga Chapova; 64–65, 66, 102–103: FotoHelin; 67: Dragon Images; 68–69: shapovalphoto; 80, 88: Anna Ok; 81 bottom: Alice Tsygankova; 83: Cat_arch_angel; 87 bottom: Lukas Gojda; 89: triocean; 90: Natalia_Grabovskaya; 98, 153: LightField Studios; 106: MaksymKarpenko21; 118: shinshila; 122: MarcoFood; 128: Elena11; 135: Momentum studio; 138–139: P-fotography, 146: Sea Wave; 147: Juice Flair; 150: cosminbuse; 162: Anna Bortnikova; 163: Todd Maughan; 166 top, 167: Olinda; 166 bottom: Scisetti Alfio; 173: Nikolaeva Galina; 174: catalina.m; 180–181: polinaloves; 183: Pixel-Shot; 192: Gaston Cerliani; 199: Agnes Kantaruk

The following images are from iStockphoto.com: Back cover, 10–11: Sergey Kirsanov; 2–3: globalmoments; 13: klenova; 17: marilyna; 20: SStajic; 21: Miriam Cerezo Garcia; 42–43: kerdkanno; 47: Nopparat Promtha; 48: Epitavi; 49: Tetiana Kolubai; 50 top, 55, 194: Almaje; 50 bottom: bonchan; 51: marrakeshh; 56: LightFieldStudios; 58: Kisa_Markiza; 59: Milena Khosroshvili; 60: MilenaKatzer; 61: elenafetisova; 72, 152 top: Plateresca; 73, 123: ronstik; 76, 77, 203: Anna-Ok; 81 top, 159: Elenathewise; 82: Svetlana Gustova; 84:shronagasukujira; 85: Madeleine_Steinbach; 87 top: Anna Kim; 93 bottom: Daria Doroshchuk; 97: cherrycake; 107, 115, 156–157, 178: Helin Loik-Tomson; 111 top: Anastasiia Pokliatska; 113 top: OksanaKiian; 117 bottom: Studio Images; 120: Liliya Filakhtova; 121: Paveena Spooner; 124, 171: kazmulka; 125: triocean; 126, 149: Yana Tatevosian; 127: iprogressman; 128: Đorđe Milutinović; 132: nadisja; 133: Yuliia Bilousova; 137: Irrin0215; 142: IrinaBort; 143, 158: S847; 145: PORNCHAI SODA; 148: masalskaya; 151: Foremniakowski; 154: ALLEKO; 155: mescioglu; 160 AniphaeS; 168 top: HappyNati; 169: mythja; 186: EKramar; 189: Andres Victorero; 191: leonori; 197: Maria Tebryaeva; 198: perfectlab